"*Rebecca Sue* is a profoundly moving tribute to the resilience of family and the beauty of unguarded love. Kathleen Norris takes us into the heart of her sister Rebecca's world with sensitivity, courage, and insight, offering a deeply human story that resonates with both struggle and grace. This book is a remarkable testament to the sacred bonds that sustain us through life's most profound challenges."

John Swinton, professor in practical theology and pastoral care at the School of Divinity, History, and Philosophy at King's College at the University of Aberdeen

"Kathleen Norris has always written with embodied, honest, human faith. In *Rebecca Sue*, Norris brings her insight into the human condition to her relationship with her disabled younger sister. The result is an invitation for all readers to discover their own humanity and to glimpse the hidden hand of God in all things."

Amy Julia Becker, author of *To Be Made Well* and *A Good and Perfect Gift*

"Kathleen Norris turns the story of her sister Becky into one of the most memorable eulogies you'll ever hear—loving, honest, sacred. With vulnerability, humor, and the depth of spiritual insight we've come to expect from Norris, this account of her sister's life made me want to read her books all over again."

Steven Purcell, executive director of Laity Lodge and author of *Even Among These Rocks*

"Kathleen Norris doesn't shy away from the unresolved histories and social norms that shaped her life with a disabled sibling or from the mix of ordinary difficulties, earned insight, and unexpected grace that arise from conditions of human needfulness. Readers will find some of their own stories echoed here, as Norris plainly and elegantly recounts, holds open, and reconsiders her own."

Sara Hendren, author of *What Can a Body Do?* and associate professor of art, design, and architecture at Northeastern University

REBECCA SUE

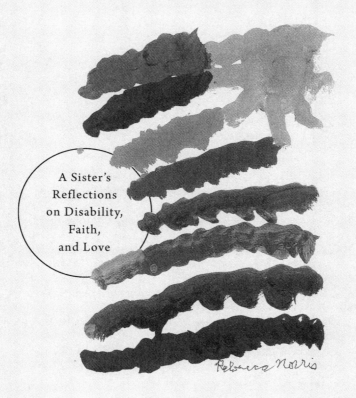

A Sister's
Reflections
on Disability,
Faith,
and Love

Rebecca Norris

KATHLEEN NORRIS

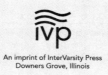

An imprint of InterVarsity Press
Downers Grove, Illinois

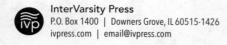

InterVarsity Press
P.O. Box 1400 | Downers Grove, IL 60515-1426
ivpress.com | email@ivpress.com

InterVarsity Press® is the publishing division of InterVarsity Christian Fellowship/USA®. For more information, visit intervarsity.org.

Scripture quotations, unless otherwise noted, are from the New Revised Standard Version, Updated Edition. Copyright © 2021 National Council of Churches of Christ in the United States of America. Used by permission. All rights reserved worldwide.

Scripture quotations from Psalms are from *The Psalms: An Inclusive Language Version Based on the Grail Translation from the Hebrew* (Chicago: GIA Publications, 1983).

Becky's letter in the chapter "I Feel Hurt Because You Wrote a Book and I Didn't" first appeared in *The Cloister Walk* (New York: Riverhead Books, 1996) in the chapter "Borderline."

While any stories in this book are true, some names and identifying information may have been changed to protect the privacy of individuals.

Published in association with The Bindery Agency, www.TheBinderyAgency.com.

The publisher cannot verify the accuracy or functionality of website URLs used in this book beyond the date of publication.

Cover design: Faceout Studio, Spencer Fuller
Interior design: Jeanna Wiggins
Cover and interior rainbow image: Rebecca Norris
Photo of Rebecca Norris on cover by Kathleen Norris

ISBN 978-1-5140-1140-9 (print) | ISBN 978-1-5140-1141-6 (digital)

Printed in the United States of America ⊗

Library of Congress Cataloging-in-Publication Data
A catalog record for this book is available from the Library of Congress.

32 31 30 29 28 27 26 25 | 13 12 11 10 9 8 7 6 5 4 3 2 1

FOR MY
PARENTS,

*John H. and
Lois T. Norris*

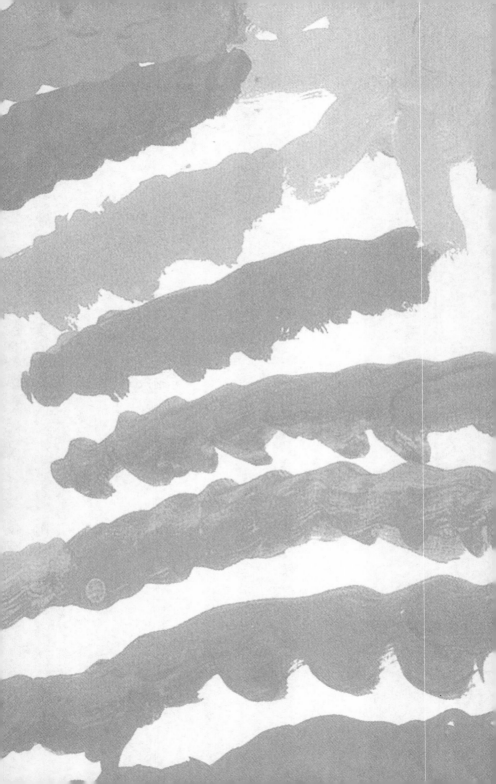

CONTENTS

NOTE TO THE READER   1

BECKY'S QUESTIONS   3

PART 1: "WILL I ALWAYS BE SLOW?"

The Rough-and-Tumble
of Family Life   9

A Good Balance   14

To Hawaii, 1959   16

Defensive Wounds   19

"You Can't Hit Me,
I'm Retarded!"   22

"Monster Mash"   23

The Beach Boys   25

Virginia Beach:
A Mellaril Haze   27

"It's All Happening
in Love with Me"   30

PART 2: "HOW DO YOU KNOW WHEN YOU'RE IN LOVE?"

"I Am in Deep Love"   35

Tora, Tora, Tora   38

"I Know How You Feel About It"   39

"I Try to Be Myself
and Not Anybody Else"   40

"I Am a Slow Learn"   44

Assessment   47

"I Am Trying to Play It Cool"   48

"They Try to Get Me Drunk"   52

The Mary of Egypt Connection   54

"I Am Having Problems
Seeing Eye to Eye with Men"   56

"It Seems like I Don't Like
the Men Who Like Me"   58

PART 3: "WHAT CAN I DO TO BE GOOD ENOUGH TO DEVELOP SKILLS?"

"A Big Poodle in the Dog House"   63

"I Try to Change for a New Me"   65

The Finder of Lost Things   68

"I Want to Change but
Am Afraid of Change"   71

"I Feel Lost Again"   73

Not Stoicism but Stability   76

"All My Dreams Get Sunk"   77

Part 4: "What Does 'Being Dependent' Mean?"

"I Know God Has a Plan for Me" 81

"If I Stay with the Family
I'll Be a Failure" 85

Mrs. R. 87

A Haunting 88

"Becky Says You're
Getting a Divorce" 92

"Please Don't Ask Me
About My Group Home" 94

"I Have a Hard Time
Loving Myself" 97

"I Can Only Change Me" 99

"I Passed the Drunk Test!" 101

Part 5: "What Will Happen to Me If You, Dad, and Mom Get Sick?"

"I Feel Hurt Because You
Wrote a Book and I Didn't" 105

"You Should Write a
Book About Me" 107

The Writer in the Family 109

Ho'omalimali 111

"I Was Praying for That" 113

"I Don't Want Mom
or Dad to Die" 115

"I'm Acting like a Child,
and I Don't Know Why" 116

Misfits 119

"I Guess This Is What It
Means to Be Bipolar" 121

"I'll Be Fine. I Have a
Positive Attitude" 123

"I Think You're Right" 126

Part 6: "It's Important to Be the Right Kind of Person"

"A Hugging Church" 131

"I Know Now People Live and Die" 133

"I Need to Spread My Wings" 135

"She Appears Older than
Her Stated Age" 137

"No One Loves You;
You Should Just Die" 140

Vows 142

"A Swan, and Not
the Ugly Duckling" 144

Phone Hugs 145

"Manicky" 149

"I Feel OK About Her Going" 152

"I Tell Them All About It" 154

Holy Week 156

Part 7: "Here We Go Again"

"She's a Mother Hen and I'm Fed Up with Her"	163
"I Wish I Could Be like Him"	165
What I Owe to Joseph Gordon-Levitt	168
"A Freak in This World"	170
"I Like It Here"	174
"Here We Go Again"	176
"The Divine Presence Is Everywhere"	178
Daisy	181
The Color Artist	183
"Thank You for Telling Me"	185

Part 8: "I Bet I Can Have Dessert Now"

"I'm Afraid That I'll Die Alone"	189
"I Bet I Can Have Dessert Now"	192
"Does She Have Faith?"	195
Rebecca Sue Norris: Medications as of April 2013	197
"We Learn a Lot About Love"	198
"I Have the Cutest Doctor, and He Surfs!"	201
Communion	203
"I Hate My Symptoms"	205
To God's Kingdom	206
"She Was Still Able to Be Herself"	208
Tulips	210
"I Am the Butterfly, Spread the Wings"	213
"Tabitha, Get Up"	214
The Perfect Thing to Say	216
Like a Child at Home	217
"It Was like She Took All the Light with Her"	219
Becky's Birds	221
The Gospel According to Rebecca	222
"And I Will Raise Them Up"	225
Iron Man 3	226

Acknowledgments	227

NOTE TO THE READER

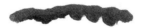

THROUGHOUT THIS BOOK, Becky's letters are presented as she wrote them, with no corrections made of her occasional misspellings or odd grammatical constructions. She used the language of her times regarding developmental and ability differences. Although many of those terms have been rightly set aside, they are the words Becky used, and I retained them.

Also be aware that this book includes mentions and descriptions of the effects of sexual assault and abuse, compulsive sexual behavior, disability, mental illness, medical issues, and death.

BECKY'S QUESTIONS

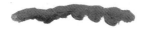

*Children who suffer from perinatal brain injury often deal
with the dramatic consequences of this misfortune for the rest of their lives.
Despite the severe clinical and socioeconomic significance,
no effective clinical strategies have yet been developed
to counteract this condition.**

WORDS SUCH AS HANDICAPPED, *disabled,* or *differently abled* are treacherous, as they allow us to label people in ways that ignore the full humanity of the person we're attempting to describe. We so often diminish people who don't fit the norm; when we see someone in a wheelchair, we're more likely to address the person tending them instead of the person sitting in the chair.

My sister Rebecca had perinatal hypoxia, but I knew and loved her as my little sister long before I heard that term applied to her. As Becky became a toddler, our parents noted that her development was not like that of my older brother and me. But that mattered less to all of us than the fact that we enjoyed the company of a lively little person, who in an atmosphere of familial love and support was developing a strong personality.

It is my intent in this book to present Rebecca Sue as a person in full. I'll begin by having her speak for herself. In going through my parents'

---

* Richard Berger, MD, Yves Garnier, MD, and Arne Jensen, MD, "Perinatal Brain Damage: Underlying Mechanisms and Neuroprotective Strategies," *Journal of the Society for Gynecologic Investigation* 9, no. 6 (November/December 2002).

correspondence after their deaths, I found that they had saved the list of questions Becky sent them when she was a teenager enrolled in a special education program at a public high school in California in the late 1960s:

Will I always be slow?

How did it happen?

What will happen to me if you, Dad, and Mom, get sick?

I'm trying to learn how to accept being slow.

What can I do to be good enough to develop skills and get real good at something?

What are academic subjects?

I'm afraid to go into crowds among strangers, where I might say the wrong thing or do something dumb.

How can a person look smarter?

Wouldn't it be great if they invent a pill someday to help people like me get smarter?

It's important to be the right kind of person. It's more important to be dependable and kind than to be smart.

What does "being dependent" mean?

How do you know when you're in love?

I'm cheating on my math.

Are others in my family slow in anything?

Why did it have to be me?

Why didn't you and mommy do something about me earlier?

These questions strike me as a perfect expression of who Becky was: her brain was damaged at birth but she was intelligent enough to know what had happened to her. Hearing words like *slow* and *dependent* applied to her and wondering what they meant. A lifelong obsession with romantic love and the search for a long-term relationship. And always that nagging "Why did it have to be me?" that sometimes led her to resent me and her other siblings.

We were a churchgoing family, with my mother raised a Presbyterian and my father descended from a long line of Methodist pastors. We didn't talk much about religion, but it was an essential part of our lives. To a large extent, because Dad was a choir director, hymns were the music of our lives. I grew up believing in the adage that when you sing you're praying twice.

In extended visits to our grandparents when I was a child, I became aware that our grandmothers provided two distinct ways of expressing the Christian faith. On our father's side, Beatrice Norris, who had met her husband at a revival meeting, felt compelled to ask other people if they had been saved. On our mother's side, Charlotte Totten had a quiet, rock-solid faith and was treasured by the women of her church for the Bible studies she offered at their meetings. Both women were uncommonly compassionate and generous, and gave credit to God for any good they were able to do in their lives.

Maybe it's the poet in me, but my favorite description of how God works in us comes in Mark 4:26-27: "The kingdom of God is as if someone would scatter seed on the ground and would sleep and rise night and day, and the seed would sprout and grow, he does not know how." When I think of my grandmothers and my parents and siblings, I see lives that express God's hidden power, described in Ephesians 3:20 as "the power at work within us" that "is able to accomplish abundantly far more than all we can ask or imagine." This feels especially true of my sister Rebecca, and I hope this book will reveal how God worked in her life, despite the daunting array of physical and mental obstacles she faced. Many people would have been driven to despair. But Becky held on; she had faith that God had something better in store for her.

If Becky taught me much about the hidden power of faith, she also taught me a lot about intelligence and the many forms it can take. She was an astute judge of people's character but couldn't solve a simple math problem. Her confession "I'm cheating on my math" makes me laugh; math anxiety is one of the many things Rebecca and I had in common. We shared a physical awkwardness and dislike of crowds and resisted taking escalators. We both believed in the power of story and felt compelled to write in order to make sense of the world. But I'm getting ahead of myself. I need to start at the beginning.

PART ONE

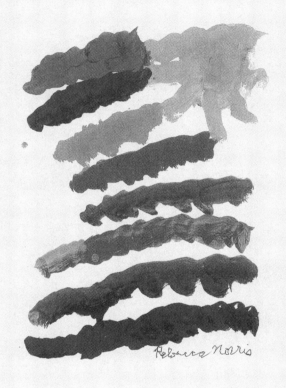

"Will I Always Be Slow?"

THE ROUGH-AND-TUMBLE
OF FAMILY LIFE

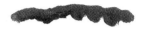

I COULD SAY THAT I GREW UP in a family with a special-needs child; but that doesn't begin to tell the story. Becky was simply one of us. In 1952, when I was five and my brother was nine, our mother went to the hospital to deliver a baby and came home with our sister Rebecca Sue. All the talk about a new baby and my becoming a big sister had excited me, but I was disappointed at my first sight of Becky. She cried a lot and had a wrinkly face, as red as an apple. I didn't understand why the grownups cooed over her, praising her dark eyes and abundant head of hair.

It was years before I heard the dire stories about Becky's birth at Bethesda Naval Hospital: how my mother had been in labor for nearly forty hours, and this being the early 1950s, the nurses had been instructed not to let the baby come until a doctor was present. My mother had been overdosed with drugs that made it more difficult for her to push when required. She knew that things were not right; she'd been through labor before, with my brother and me. During the ordeal she heard one doctor say to another, "You got yourself into this mess; let's see you get yourself out."

Mom often expressed concern over how slow Becky was to grab for things, vocalize, and walk. Becky never did learn to crawl, but she developed an impressive ability to scoot like a little rocket around the house, clinging to a bit of blue blanket that she called her "mine." This became a model for how Becky responded to obstacles. When she couldn't do things "the right way," she invented a way that suited her. We had this in common. When I took a required typing class in high school, I struggled to follow the rules and afterward developed a typing style that is mine alone.

My parents suspected that damage had been done during my sister's birth, but doctors were not forthcoming with a diagnosis. When Becky was four they advised my parents to put her in an institution. Mom and Dad discussed this with me and my brother, John, and we all agreed that it was unthinkable to let Becky go; she was part of our family.

As a child I didn't think of my family as different from any other. We kids had our squabbles in the rough-and-tumble of family life, and Becky was just a part of that. She was game to join us and the neighborhood children in playing hide-and-seek or running from imaginary elephants or wild horses.

The family had left Washington, DC, when my father, who had been an assistant conductor and orchestrator for the US Navy Band, was assigned to lead the band at the Great Lakes Naval Training Center outside Chicago. In the early 1950s we were living in a house in Beach Park, between Waukegan and Zion, one of several new homes in a nascent suburb; across the street a farmer tended a large cornfield.

There was a small slope in the front yard and during our first winter, John figured that with enough snow you could get a decent sled ride. One day he and Becky tried their luck. Becky was excited about sledding with her big brother, and I was content to cheer them on. We sometimes failed to grasp that Becky had difficulty understanding practical realities, like the importance of having the sled go straight down the hill and not sideways.

The sled was heavy. It had been our mother's when she was a child, and we had brought it from her hometown in South Dakota the summer before. Becky's skinny little arm got stuck in the wrong place and she yelled, sounding more surprised than in pain. John and I knew Becky was injured, but she wanted to try another ride. When we finally got her into the house and Mom got Becky's jacket off, one arm was hanging at an odd angle. Clearly, there was a broken bone, but all Becky said was, "Mommy; my arm hurts."

Becky was more accident prone than the rest of us. Once when we were visiting our grandparents in South Dakota, John, Becky, and I were taking turns riding a neighbor's old, gentle horse. While Becky was riding, the horse suddenly knelt and rolled over her. You don't realize how enormous a horse is until you see your little sister disappear underneath it. When the horse rose again, Becky stood up on her own and walked toward us. Our grandfather, a physician, examined her on the spot. She wasn't hurt or even upset.

Our mother didn't know what to make of two daughters who were notably awkward. She enrolled me in an excruciating "tumbling class," where I consistently failed to execute somersaults and simple dance routines. With Becky, she didn't even try, except that she insisted that all her children take swimming lessons at the local YMCA. Her biggest concern about Becky was her lack of common sense, and Becky did give us scares from time to time. Our house had a basement that Becky was not allowed to enter unless someone accompanied her on the stairs. The steps came straight down from the kitchen, but near the end you had to take a sharp turn just right, or risk falling onto the concrete floor. I enjoyed playing with my toys in the basement but found the stairs frightening, and descended them with caution.

Once when Becky was given permission to go downstairs to play with John, she became so excited that she took the stairs too fast and began to tumble. Mom had been following her but was unable to get hold of her in the narrow stairwell. John caught Becky in his arms. He says it was fairly easy, as she was a bean pole in those days, but he marvels that she was so eager to play that she was nonchalant about the danger she'd been in.

I have a similar memory. When my elementary school band marched in a parade at a Chicago-area amusement park, we were rewarded with passes for free rides. As Becky and I explored the park, we bypassed the roller coaster, as we'd learned that it would make us sick. But a ride on two-seater boats with large rubber bumpers looked promising. You steered the boat around a pool and deliberately crashed into the other boats.

I sat in front and steered and Becky sat in back, laughing happily until she apparently decided that she wanted to stop. If she said anything, I didn't hear it over the noise of the boat motors and people shouting. It was a change in that sound—people screaming, sounding panicked—that alerted me: Becky had stood up and was in danger of falling into the water. People stopped their boats until I got Becky to sit down. As I drove our boat to the exit, Becky began to cry. I tried to reassure her that everything would be okay; I can still see that dark, greasy water.

The family's biggest change came in 1954, when my mother became pregnant. My parents believed that Becky's disability had been the result of medical error but were concerned this new baby might also be "slow." They needn't have worried. When Charlotte arrived in early 1955, she was so robust the obstetrician commented that she might as well walk home. She proved to be mentally and physically agile, early to crawl, walk, and form words. She also developed a forceful personality and could outdo any of us in stubbornness.

Mom felt that Becky was fortunate to have a sister just three years younger because in attempting to keep up with her, Becky developed skills she might otherwise have lacked. She learned to play jacks, for example, which I never mastered. And Charlotte's facility with speech challenged Becky to up her game. The most important thing Charlotte did was to tell Becky no. Being so close in age to Becky was hard on her, and she learned early on to protect herself. She was quicker than the rest of us to refuse to indulge Becky because of her disability.

I was five years older than Becky, eight years older than Charlotte, and that was enough for me to often regard them both as nuisances. If I held myself as above their more childish pursuits, like playing with Barbie dolls, it didn't mean that I loved them any less. I just became a little less likely to show it. As we all matured, both of my sisters provided me with plenty of surprises, becoming people I not only loved but came to admire.

A GOOD BALANCE

As busy as our parents were, they were a source of stability and security. We ate a home-cooked dinner nearly every night, during which time the television—then a novelty—was turned off so we could visit. Dad usually had an after-work martini, and we drank water or milk with our meals. Soda was reserved for special occasions like birthdays or the rare treat of eating at McDonald's, which had opened in Waukegan in 1955.

Church was always a part of our life. Dad's father and grandfather had been Methodist ministers, and his ancestors had pastored churches in England as far back as the late fifteenth century. My grandmother Charlotte Totten was solidly Presbyterian; even as a child I recognized that she had an unshakable moral compass. Her husband Frank Totten, a physician, supported the church financially but mostly left religion up to his wife. My siblings and I were baptized by our Grandfather Norris, and when we were older confirmation was a given. While Becky liked the kindly pastor who taught the class, she didn't pay much attention to its content. But she was thrilled to received her own copy of the Bible. I could sympathize; I'd long loved the stories in the Bible, but memorizing a catechism left me cold.

Photographs depict my sisters and me posing in outfits that Grandmother Totten had bought us for Easter Sunday, complete with hats, little purses, lacy socks, and Mary Jane shoes. At Christmas we sat in front of a tinsel-laden tree to open gifts. In one photo I'm grinning as I show off a new doll, with one hand resting on a rocking horse that

Santa had brought my younger sisters. Becky is perched uneasily on it, looking down with an anxious expression, as if she's trying to figure out how to stay seated on something so unsteady. Instinctively, I'm trying to help her keep her balance.

When I think of the balancing act my parents performed with four children, jobs, and civic commitments, I wonder if they weren't uniquely suited for the task. My father was born in West Virginia in 1916 and at four years of age moved to South Dakota with his family of six. In South Dakota two girls and a boy were born. As the Methodist church then moved pastors every two years, my dad lived in De Smet, Colome, Salem, Mitchell, Kimball, Groton, Faith, Hot Springs, and Murdo, where he graduated from high school in 1935. My mother's home life had been stable by comparison. She was born in Lemmon, South Dakota, in 1917, and lived in the same house from infancy through high school.

My parents brought to their marriage the fervor, impulsiveness, and good humor of the Norris clan and the quiet piety, restraint, and a combination of realism and optimism that marked the Tottens. I believe that this marriage of opposites gave our family a good balance between stability and openness to change. It may also have given us an advantage when it came to living with Becky. A special-needs child can place considerable strain on a family. But we took Becky's difficulties in stride, at least during her childhood.

TO HAWAII, 1959

SOMETIME IN THE 1950s I heard my dad say to my mom, after returning from a dinner party, "I've never been so bored in my life." I didn't understand that: my mother had been looking forward to that party, as it gave her a chance to dress up, and I had watched her engage in the ritual she called "putting on her face," applying powder, rouge, Love That Red lipstick, and White Shoulders perfume. It all seemed exciting to me.

Dad's restlessness with suburban life may have been one reason he convinced my mother to uproot the family and move to the territory of Hawaii when the Navy band director's job at Pearl Harbor opened up. He had first gone to Hawaii in 1944, when the Navy sent him to play in its band there and also perform in the free concerts offered by the military during the war. He had loved Hawaii. And one cold morning when the family car wouldn't start, it triggered his desire to return. He traveled to Washington, DC, to request a transfer, taking his ukulele to press the point, and soon received orders to report to Pearl.

After the moving van left with our household goods, we loaded ourselves, luggage, and camping equipment into our station wagon with a U-Haul trailer and left for the West Coast, stopping in Iowa and South Dakota to say goodbye to relatives. Becky and I enjoyed looking out the car window at the passing scenery but endured much teasing from John and Charlotte, as we both got motion sickness.

I was excited at the idea of crossing the Rockies but had never before been in the mountains. As Dad drove higher and higher on the winding roads, one look down terrified me so much I buried my head in a pillow. Becky did much better, content to look at the spectacular scenery. That characterized her; a serene faith that in the face of danger everything would be fine. While she seldom spoke of God, I believe she'd taken her Sunday school lessons to heart and was more certain than I that God would always be looking out for us.

My experience of God on that trip was one of awe, waking in a tent one bright, chilly morning in Yellowstone National Park to find a clear cerulean sky above, and an inch of snow on the ground that had fallen overnight. It was the middle of May. As we drove through Nevada, I was delighted to see the desert in bloom.

We arrived in San Francisco with wrinkled clothes and dirty faces and went to a large downtown hotel with our voucher from the Navy. Mother was embarrassed when we walked past people in fancy evening dress, but Becky and Charlotte, enthralled by the posh hotel lobby, were oblivious to the disapproving stares. The next day we moved to an old army post, Fort Mason in the Marina District, to await our flight to Honolulu. We took long walks along the bay, stretching our legs after days of riding in a car. We enjoyed being tourists in the city, and John and I looked forward to riding the famous cable cars. Charlotte was just four, but she loved them. As often happened with Becky, the idea was more appealing than the reality. The clanging bells so disturbed her that she became weepy and clung to Mom, insisting on sitting on her lap.

On arriving at Travis Air Force Base for our flight, we boarded a four-propeller military plane, a Lockheed Constellation. It was the first flight for all of us except our dad, who'd flown on planes during the US Navy's Shipmate Variety tours in the mid-1950s. It was a long haul, well over eleven hours in a plane whose ventilation system wasn't working well. A few hours into the flight we were provided with a dispiriting box lunch of cold fried chicken, an apple, and a candy bar. We children were too restless to sleep, and our parents had to endure endless versions of "Are we there yet?"

We arrived at Hickam Air Force Base a little after one on a June morning. The air that greeted us as we descended from the plane on metal stairs was warm, moist, and scented with flowers. Mom said she felt like she was in a steam bath. We were housed overnight in a barracks on base. I shared a room with my sisters; our beds were equipped with scratchy wool blankets. Not long after I got to sleep I was awakened by screams. Charlotte had dared to venture alone to a bathroom down the hall and encountered a "B-52," the local term for an American cockroach, three inches long and nearly an inch wide. It took my mother and father some time to get to her and calm her down. I wondered if Air Force personnel used to the roar of fighter jets had been astonished at how loud a little girl's screams could be in the middle of the night. Becky slept through it all.

DEFENSIVE WOUNDS

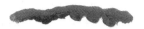

WHEN WE ARRIVED, Hawaii was about to become a state, and we all went to see Dad's Navy band parade down Kalakaua Avenue in the statehood celebrations. As they settled into Navy housing, Mom and Dad prepared to enroll their children in public schools and discovered a faulty education system with an entrenched and inflexible bureaucracy. My brother, about to enter his junior year of high school, was interested in a career in science, but the school he was assigned to offered no chemistry classes, and my parents were told he could not transfer to another school.

The textbook for my seventh grade class was the same one I'd used in sixth grade in Illinois, and Mom and Dad suggested to the school administration that I be allowed to skip a grade. The refusal came with the comment that if I knew the book so well, I could help the teacher. Mom and Dad did what would have been unthinkable to them in the past and applied for scholarships to a private school for my brother and me. But there were no alternatives for Becky. She attended a public school that was ill-equipped to work with a child with brain damage.

My parents had Becky tested at Tripler Army Hospital and at last received a name for her condition: *perinatal hypoxia*. She had been deprived of oxygen at a critical time during her birth. According to the National Institutes of Health, perinatal hypoxia and perinatal asphyxia account for a third of neonatal deaths. My sister could have died in the process of being born. Side effects of perinatal hypoxia can include cerebral palsy, epilepsy, severe seizures, cognitive disabilities, and behavioral disorders. Becky had the last two in spades but was mercifully spared the others.

It is difficult for me to imagine what a torment it was for Becky to leave a familial atmosphere of love and understanding and enter Chester W. Nimitz Elementary School, where in 1959 "special education" was a foreign concept. Every weekday my sister Becky was expected to attend a school where she was ridiculed by other students for being "stupid" and treated with indifference or worse by teachers who had little idea of how to work with students who had special needs. Becky told us that she tried to be invisible in the classroom so that the teacher wouldn't call on her. She was getting Fs in every subject, even art, which we knew she loved.

I'm proud of my sister for rebelling against this mistreatment by refusing to go to school. One day she threw a tantrum so severe that even the school principal couldn't get her out of the family car. Becky knew that she was being badly treated by her school, and she wasn't going down without a fight.

When our parents took Becky out of school, the state threatened to sue. In a compromise, Mom and Dad were allowed to hire a tutor. At the first session, Becky surprised the tutor by being unusually demonstrative, hugging the woman and saying, "I like you." She was appalled that Becky's teachers had been passing her to the next grade without teaching her basics she was capable of learning. Becky's language skills quickly improved with her guidance. But while she could sometimes get Becky to grasp a mathematic concept and successfully work out a simple problem, at their next session she'd have to start over, as Becky would not have retained the information.

Becky thrived under this woman's attention and eventually was able to return to school. But a rudimentary special education program still did not serve her well. One teacher put her special ed students to work cleaning the classroom. At another school near Pearl Harbor, two abandoned buildings were designated for special ed students but were so rundown that the Navy Officers' Wives Club donated supplies so that my father and volunteers could paint them and make repairs. Becky's teacher was well-meaning but only semiqualified. The emotional damage my sister suffered in those years left her with defensive wounds that she carried for the rest of her life.

"YOU CAN'T HIT ME, I'M RETARDED!"

BECKY DISCOVERED THAT this line doesn't work with sisters, especially one who has witnessed you writing on a cement-block wall with her first lipstick. She was jealous because I had a lipstick and she didn't, and knew that what she was doing was wrong. I knew that hitting her would get me into serious trouble, but I was outraged and swatted at Becky with a handy book of sheet music. We yelled at each other until our exasperated mom intervened.

Growing up with Becky, it was always a challenge to distinguish between what she needed to be held accountable for and what she couldn't help doing due to her disability. That fine line was constantly in flux, which kept me on my toes.

For years afterward Becky would recount this story, telling people what she had said to me: "You can't hit me, I'm retarded." This was Becky in a nutshell: aware of her difference just enough to take advantage of it.

"MONSTER MASH"

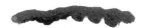

IF YOU MENTION THE 1960s novelty song "Monster Mash" to my siblings, you're likely to get a groan. When Becky came home after a day at school, she would retreat to her room, throw her books against the wall, and scream out her frustrations. In that room, unlike at school, Becky was in control.

When a novelty song titled "Monster Mash" became a hit, Becky played the 45 repeatedly on a small portable record player every afternoon. She was then sharing a room with Charlotte, who usually played outdoors with friends or helped Mom in the kitchen while Becky was ranting.

I had my own room next door and got used to doing homework to the beat of "Monster Mash," and hearing Becky shout at people who weren't there. I didn't complain, as I realized that Becky needed this time to vent, rehashing the day and responding to people who had called her "stupid" or "retarded." She'd been made to feel like a monster, and playing that song was the way she had found to reset her life and gain the strength to face the next day.

One day, as I heard Becky stomping around and scolding someone who had scorned her, I realized how alike we were. I too was a social outcast and needed solitude to recover from a day with snobbish classmates. And I also inflicted my favorite music on my family. Most mornings before I left for school I sat in the living room and listened to Rossini's *La forza del destino*, Barber's *Adagio for Strings*, or Bob Dylan songs.

My survival methods were quieter than Becky's. I kept my dialogues with others in my head. But hearing Becky play "Monster Mash" every afternoon, I began to see that she and I shared an emotional vulnerability. She had the burden of brain damage; I had the burden of being adept at keeping my inner turmoil to myself.

THE BEACH BOYS

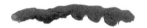

WE ALL KNEW THAT LOUD NOISES and being in crowds upset Becky. In the early 1960s, Dad played cello in the Honolulu Symphony, and we often went to the concerts. They performed at an outdoor venue, the Waikiki Shell, and we'd bring blankets and sit on the lawn. One year, when Tchaikovsky's *1812 Overture* was on the program, we sat farther back than usual and warned Becky about the cannons. Even so, their sound made her stiffen; she put her hands to her ears and began to cry.

I was apprehensive when one day in 1963 I was more or less ordered by my parents to take Becky to an afternoon concert by the Beach Boys at a small outdoor venue on a military base. Becky had said that she wanted to go, but I worried about how she would react to the amplified music. And I was resentful, not wanting to sit through the mindless music that my more popular peers enjoyed. I took pride in my eclectic tastes: give me the Bach cello suites, Bix Beiderbecke, or Frank Sinatra's *Only the Lonely* album any day. But not the Beach Boys.

I learned a great lesson that day, and not just because I enjoyed the Beach Boys far more than I expected to, and more than I was willing to admit at the time. Like many adolescents, I was selfish and self-absorbed, but when I put aside my own desires and did this simple thing for my sister, I received far more than I could have imagined. Becky's social life was even more constrained than mine, and it was lovely to see how delighted she was to be attending a rock concert like any preteen girl.

The Beach Boys had an opening act. It was a singer I hadn't heard of, but his voice stunned me into submission. All the petty annoyances of the event—the noise; the crowd; the long, hot afternoon—evaporated as he sang. It was Roy Orbison, and I can now claim that I have heard an angel sing.

VIRGINIA BEACH:
A MELLARIL HAZE

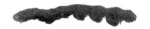

IN 1965, THE NAVY ASSIGNED my father to teach at the Navy School of Music in Virginia, and although we were reluctant to leave Hawaii, it seemed like a good time for the family to make the transition. My brother had just graduated from the University of Hawaii with a degree in mathematics, and I had just graduated from high school in Honolulu. I'd be attending Bennington College in the fall and liked the idea of my family being close, a train ride away rather than in far-off Honolulu.

For our return to the US mainland, the Navy sent us on a luxury passenger ship, the *Lurline*. On that five-day voyage I learned how the Pacific got its name: the ocean was often as still as a pond. Dad was invited to play with the musicians on board, sitting in with his cornet as they played for passengers in the evenings. My mother enjoyed dressing up for dinner. My brother played shuffleboard, and on most afternoons I settled into a chair and read, alternating *Moby Dick* with James Bond novels. Charlotte, age ten, befriended a boy her age who was traveling with his grandmother, and the two of them became inseparable.

We all tried to keep an eye on Becky, who was nearly thirteen. But she resented being treated like a child, and we couldn't protect her from being sexually molested by a steward, who no doubt saw my sister—awkward, shy, socially isolated—as easy prey. As is often the case when a child suffers sexual abuse, she told no one about it at the time and didn't fully understand what had happened to her. It was years before my parents learned about the abuse from one of Becky's psychiatrists, and it wasn't until I read the notes from her longtime counselor that I realized how much this horrific event had haunted her and shaped her perspective on her body and relationships with men.

But Becky seemed fine at the time, and after a night of rolling seas as we approached San Francisco, we disembarked and said goodbye to my brother, who was heading for training as a Peace Corps volunteer. The rest of us headed up the coast in our Volkswagen camper, driving through the redwood and sequoia forests. We spent an extra night at one national park because we'd camped at a lovely site by a stream and wanted more time for walks through the enormous trees. When Becky got too close to the water's edge and fell into the stream, Dad quickly got her out of the shallow water. Heading north, we camped out in provincial parks across Canada, passing through the splendors of Banff and Lake Louise. Then we crossed into South Dakota to visit relatives before continuing on to the East Coast.

After the family settled into Navy housing in Virginia Beach, Mom obtained a job teaching in a preschool that was part of the new Head Start program for disadvantaged children. The school often received bomb threats, as it was one of the few integrated schools in the area. Along with his Navy duties, Dad played cello in the Norfolk Symphony. Charlotte's outgoing personality brought her many friends and an active social life. Becky was no doubt jealous, and this, along with her experience of abuse, made her an easy mark for two brothers in the neighborhood who engaged Becky in their games of sexual play and petty crimes.

Mom and Dad often gave Charlotte the unenviable task of looking after her older sister, and she believes they had little idea of what Becky was up to. She once had to drag Becky out of the bedroom of one of the brothers, while the other tried to grab and assault her. Even after nearly sixty years she recalls his name—and how surprised he was that she fought back so fiercely he had to let her go.

I was in college but lived with the family over Christmas, summer vacations, and for one Bennington nonresident term. When Bennington students left in December, they didn't return until early March; over the winter they worked in jobs or internships. One year I was a kindergarten aide at a Quaker elementary school, another racially integrated school in Norfolk.

Becky's school experience in Virginia was another miserable one. She was enrolled in a special education program and my parents liked her teacher, but the students were routinely bullied by other kids at the school. Her teacher felt that Becky needed counseling, and Mom and Dad engaged a psychiatrist, who prescribed Becky's first psychotropic drugs. Once when I was home from college and suffering from insomnia, I took one of my sister's Mellaril tablets. It knocked me out for over twelve hours, and even after I woke I felt groggy. Becky was taking two to four Mellaril a day. She was fourteen years old.

Mellaril was a brand name of an antipsychotic drug thioridazine, which was often prescribed for schizophrenics. I'm not sure if Becky had been misdiagnosed as schizophrenic or if the physician was using the drug to decrease abnormal excitement in the brain. But the drug dulled Becky emotionally, casting her normally vibrant personality into the shadows. While she could become overexcited and overbearing, Mom and Dad decided they'd rather have their lively daughter back, and got a second opinion. Becky was taken off Mellaril, but something else was prescribed for her. She took psychotropic drugs for the rest of her life.

After two years in Norfolk, the family made an unexpected move back to Hawaii. The man who had replaced Dad as the bandmaster at Pearl Harbor was an old friend, and one day he called my dad and said that his wife hated Hawaii and they were leaving. He asked if Dad was interested in returning, and soon the family left for Hawaii again.

"IT'S ALL HAPPENING IN LOVE WITH ME"

IN 1967, WHEN I WAS A COLLEGE JUNIOR and Becky was fifteen, my father's persistent efforts to get the Navy to take more responsibility for Becky's condition paid off when the Navy agreed to pay Becky's tuition, room, and board at the Devereux School in Santa Barbara, California. A school for young people living with emotional, behavioral, or cognitive differences, it offered resources not available in Hawaii. In his annual Christmas letter my father wrote: "At Devereux Becky finally learned that school can be a happy experience." He noted that she had found "acceptance by her peers, boy and girl friends, successes, and independence. Having Devereux and Becky find each other has been the happiest experience of the year for us all." When he sent Becky blank cassette tapes, she was so excited about reporting on her life at the school that she'd talk until the tape ran out.

Becky wrote many letters to me from Devereux, and in late December of that year I flew from Vermont, met Becky at the San Francisco airport, and we flew together to Honolulu. I was thrilled to have lined up a nonresident term job in the library of the renowned Bishop Museum. Becky didn't want to hear about that; she talked incessantly about how much she loved working on the Devereux school newspaper, conducting interviews and reporting on student council meetings and campus events. She'd discovered that she liked writing, and in one of the many letters she sent me after that Christmas, she included a poem she'd written for a class. I was touched that she had dedicated it to me:

To Kathy

It's green leaves

and white raindrops

that make my day lovely.

It's rain and thunder that make

me feel like wandering

around the sky and earth.

Blue sky and colors everywhere

it's all happening in love with me.

PART TWO

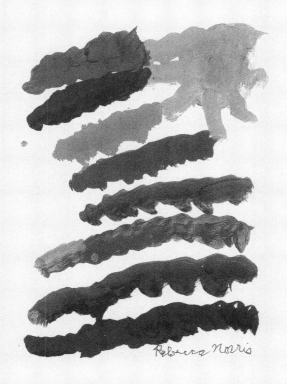

Rebecca Norris

"How Do You Know
When You're in Love?"

"I AM IN DEEP LOVE"

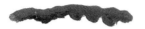

DEVEREUX AIMED TO PREPARE young people for careers, and Becky initially worked there as a cafeteria server and dishwasher. She wrote to me, "I want to work extra so I can get out faster and be able to get a job." But her being in California meant that she was going through the turmoil of adolescence away from home, and the consequences were unsettling. Becky sent this letter to our parents when she was seventeen:

> Dear Parents,
>
> . . . I am fine and hope you understand this, but you are going to be shocked. But after I finish my High School and get a job, Bill and I are going to live together and I am in real love with him and he is in love with me and he wanted to do sex with me but not all the way, but I said no because I didn't want to hurt you both cause I love my family very much and do love Bill an awful lot and now we understand a little bit about each other . . . what do you think about this? I am scared of what you might think of me but I cannot help feeling that I love him a great deal like how you love each other . . . it's exactly the same feeling about love, so please write to me cause I don't want the whole school to find out . . . I am in deep love and I am not fooling around at all. I know it is shocking news to you but that's how life is.
>
> Love, Becky

In a letter written to me on the same day, Becky expressed her concerns about how our parents would respond to her news: "I feel afraid of my own family to say I am going to get married but you always say when you are in love you will know it by feeling and I feel that it is true love but I am afraid that they won't understand about it." If this news startled me, it was because Becky had written me just a few days earlier: "I have given up on boys here cause I have about gone with everyone here and they aren't my type at all. I want a guy who is nice and a great personally and who respect me for what I am not for what I am not."

When they received the letter, Mom probably had to talk Dad out of boarding the next plane to California. Becky was adept at changing the subject whenever she found herself on shaky ground. Immediately after giving our parents the news of her impending marriage, she told them that she was nervous because she was slated to be tested to see if she'd qualify for a program called the Academy, which would involve her taking some classes at a local public high school.

Mom eventually went to California to see Becky, met her boyfriend, and learned more about the Academy. Mom felt that the transition to a more rigorous program would be difficult for Becky, but it was worth a try, as having more demanding schoolwork might make Becky less likely to focus on boys.

Writing to me, Becky said, "I finally got into a public high school and have a Special Education class for two periods. It's easy for me." She explains that when she's done with school she plans to return to Hawaii and get a job. But as usual, it's the drama of relationships that most concerns her. She writes that a girl who is her closest friend

is very mad at me and I am about to do something to myself and its really hurt inside of me. I wish you're here with me talking to her because I begin cry all nite and if I don't talk to her it will wreck this last school year and I will failure it and I don't even know what to do at all. Please write back to me about something about what you'll do about it. I am scared of it. Please help me out.

Becky

I wrote back and the situation with her friend soon resolved itself; the girl later came to visit Becky and our family in Honolulu. As for Bill, while in February Becky had believed that she was in love with him, by May she was trying to ignore him. She wrote, "I am trying to get rid of Bill but it is really hard to do when the persons here at school—got any ideas to help your sister about her big problem?" She offered this advice: "Don't get too involve with a guy if you can't trust him," adding, "I have found someone who likes me better." Bill was still on her mind, however, and in October she wrote,

Dear Kathy,

Thank you very much for your letter it really cheer me up. I was talking to Bill and he still likes me and he said I needed to change and I said I will do it. I'm trying to not make up stories about people any more. I know sometimes I act like a little kid. Do you think I really need to change for the better? I feel like I am not satisfactory with myself. So let me know when you have time to write me.

As I lived apart from Becky for years, letters became our main way of communicating, along with the occasional long-distance phone call. In Becky's letters from Devereux, themes emerge that were to recur throughout her life: a deep but unfulfilled desire to find a job that would allow her to support herself, and most of all, finding a man to love who would love her in return.

TORA, TORA, TORA

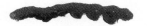

My father became a member of the Screen Actors Guild when the producers of the film *Tora, Tora, Tora* realized that the easiest way to depict a Navy band performing a flag-raising ceremony at Pearl Harbor on the morning of December 7, 1941, was to hire the US Navy Band stationed there. If you've seen the film, you've witnessed the US Pacific Fleet band playing the national anthem with my father conducting.

The director liked my dad's looks enough to give him a brief, full-face shot, which is cut when the movie appears on cable TV. But it apparently lasted long enough that he was required to join the guild. The band members were thrilled to be paid well for doing an ordinary job, and my dad used the money he earned to travel with my sister Becky to the East Coast. They visited me at Bennington in Vermont and then went to Virginia to see his mother and sister, my aunt Kathleen.

It was during my sister's visit to Bennington that I began to understand how astute Becky could be about people. She quickly sized up the married man with whom I'd been having an affair and figured out before I did that he was a habitual philanderer. I had been blinded by infatuation, but my sister was thinking more clearly. With typical candor she asked, "How can you love him, when he's married?"

During Becky's visit to Bennington I also witnessed how my sister blossomed when she encountered someone who treated her with sensitivity and respect. I introduced Becky to a classmate, an uncommonly kind woman who was planning to become a teacher. She had worked as an aide in special education classes, and on meeting Becky she immediately grasped who my sister was and what her needs were. Becky drank in the affection, and the two of them corresponded for years.

"I KNOW HOW YOU FEEL ABOUT IT"

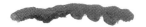

BECKY HAD BEEN WORRIED about my affair with a married man, and after I'd graduated from college and was working in New York City, I wrote and told her that he had moved on to another young woman. She responded with this advice, writing

> I know how you feel about it cause I have been in the same situation and I have said to myself there is a lot of fish in the sea. If I see someone I would like to meet I would just say HI my name is Rebecca Norris and he would tell me his name and I would ask him a question like, what kind of sports do you like? or what things do you do in your spare time? Then we would talk about it and we would first be friends. Now how does that sound?

I took comfort in her words; they were pure Becky and helped me laugh at myself. She reminded me that where love and romance were concerned, we shared a naive and idealized notion of finding a grand passion, a love that would dazzle us and sweep us off our feet. We were slow to recognize that this ideal was both unattainable and dangerous, a misdirecting of our capacity for devotion. We craved the raging emotions that came with being in love, or more accurately, being in love with love, and sought out people who were inappropriate or unattainable. It took us both a long time to comprehend that love meant committing to another person, someone who would make demands of us but also love and care for us in return.

"I TRY TO BE MYSELF AND NOT ANYBODY ELSE"

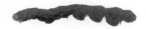

BECKY REGRESSED SEVERELY whenever she came home from Devereux. This may be a common phenomenon; young people who've tasted independence have difficulty adjusting to being under their parents' roofs again. But with Becky, every Christmas break brought extreme turmoil. Dad described one year as "the roughest ever. She has such a terrible self-image and view of the future. She spent 90 percent of her time in her room or watching TV. We couldn't even get her out of the house to go see her dad in *Tora*."

He notes that she hadn't had many close friendships at Devereux that year and that the other girls in the Academy intimidated her. "Nevertheless," he writes, "the plan is that she will return for another year, as she isn't ready to go out into the job market."

My mother sent me the school's report on Becky:

Her ability to make decisions has improved—she has matured but needs more self-confidence. She continues to need an abnormal amount of approval and praise, but has not once avoided job responsibilities by staying in bed, etc. We conclude that Becky is now ready to take the next big step:

1. After the Christmas break she should move off campus to a foster home;

2. She should continue in her present job unless a paying one comes along;

3. If she is to be successful in a job experience, then returning to Hawaii to be closer to her parents should be considered. Staying here another year in preparation might be necessary. We felt that readjustment to living with her family might be difficult, and there could be regression.

Devereux found her a volunteer job at a rehabilitation center for physically disabled children, and this inspired Becky to pay more attention to her appearance. She wrote to me, "I try to fix myself up all the time to look nice. I try to be myself and not anybody else." Adding a typical plea, she wrote, "I have two things to work on and would like your suggestions, OK? One is gossiping about others to hurt them and the other is becoming a young woman. These are the only ones I feel I need help on. Plus I whine in my voice and I try not to do it. Love Becky."

Becky's return to Honolulu for that Christmas did not go well. Dad wrote me that "Becky got off the plane mad at the whole world and started snarling about the way the school overprotects them. She had made it on her own to the Honolulu flight and was already in her seat when the 'sponsor' who was supposed to meet her and see that she made that connection finally caught up with her. Becky was embarrassed by all the unwanted attention on the plane." Typically, she nursed her anger in silence during the flight and exploded when she met her parents.

In a letter to me, Dad reports that at first Becky "wouldn't go anyplace with us—told us emphatically that she wasn't going back to Devereux. She was hard to get along with, negative about everything, and mentioned more than once that you were the only one who understood her." I phoned from New York several times to see if I could get her to voice her concerns, but Becky always said things were fine.

By Christmas Day, Becky had decided that the new situation in California would be good for her, writing to me: "I will have a great year cause I'll get a foster home and I'll be proud. I am a different person. I haven't slam any door or flip out at home. I been helping Mom clean house and started to go everywhere with everybody."

My mother sums up Becky's stay at home with typical under-statement, writing that "while we had some of our annual Christmas trauma with Becky, we lived through it, and in general she was easier to live with." Still, Becky tended to withdraw into her room, listen to the radio, and talk to herself. When Harry, a young man she'd known for years and who had always treated her well, showed up to see her, she locked herself in her room.

One year I had been able to come from New York City to be with my family at Christmas but had to return before the New Year. My dad wrote to me, "After you left Becky was depressed for a couple of days. She slept a lot, and was uncommunicative. She tried to explain that she missed you because you two think alike."

Becky had been disbelieving when I told her that I had also faced many anxieties every time I prepared to return to college after a summer break. But it became clear that Becky was at the mercy of fierce impulses that led to increasingly erratic behavior. One year Dad wrote that "when she was to fly to California, she reverted in a familiar way. When we were due to leave for the airport she was curled up in her bed in a fetal position, making animal noises and refusing to budge. I had to cancel the plane reservation and phone the school."

By that night she had become contrite and agreeable. Dad wrote that Becky had "turned 180 degrees, had done all the dishes and laundry and made the beds." He made new plane reservations, and on the way to the airport he said "she talked about her fears. 'How do you budget?' was a big one. Also she asked, 'How do you get your savings out of one bank and into another?' These things are real worries for her."

A gate agent allowed Dad to walk Becky onto the plane, and she told him, "When I get this far, I'm OK." She had calmed down: "No tears," he wrote, "and she hurried me off the plane." But he remained at the airport until her flight was airborne. "It is always an emotional experience for me," he wrote. "I watch the clock all day, and wonder where she is, how she's doing." Becky made her connecting flight in San Francisco and arrived safely at Santa Barbara, where her foster parents picked her up at the airport. They called my parents and put Becky on the phone. Dad said that she "sounded happy, and seemed to have her anxieties under control for the moment. But we know she is going to continue to be a problem we must face. She has just one more year at most at Devereux and then we'll see."

"I AM A SLOW LEARN"

BECKY WROTE TO ME that she liked her foster parents and a new counselor, stating that after talking with him she "didn't have fears about anything." She liked having her own room and declared, "I am more responsible. I go to work every day. I don't get paid but I am sticking it out. I am more depend by myself. My hair is almost down to my shoulders. But I've a problem I can't tell you. Becky."

As was often the case, the problem concerned a young man. She had allowed an attraction to become a full-blown crush, and then came on too strong, which led the boy to reject her. Her other constant concern was finding work. After I had written to suggest that she concentrate more on her schoolwork than boys she wrote: "Your letter really help me out—I am just good friends with my male friends and that's all there is. I have an interview this week to see what job will be suitable for me since I am a slow learn. Well I got to go for now. Love Becky."

Becky enjoyed working with physically disabled children and so impressed the hospital staff that they soon expanded her three days a week to five. Eventually they offered to pay her. At the end of May she wrote: "Guess what I will get paid for two hours a day at $1.35 and I get my first paid check on June 9 and I just can't believe it. It's a demanding job but I do it pretty good." When Dad visited he was impressed with how well Becky was handling such difficult work. "Her patients," he writes, "are severely deformed and dependent children. But Becky feeds, bathes, and plays with them. She's affectionate and gentle, and talks to them while she is exercising them. It's clear to everyone that she loves them. She's doing so well at this job that the staff has asked her to help train their volunteers."

Dad found that "even the kids who can't talk make happy sounds when they see Becky. Her co-workers say that she's good at seeing what needs to be done, and they intend to increase her work load to six hours a day. Also, as they are connected with an institution in Honolulu, they could arrange a job for her should she return home."

The staff told Dad that there had been some adjustment problems. When people would go about their tasks without engaging Becky in casual conversations, she thought they didn't like her. "Finally," he wrote, "she told her co-workers that she was a slow learner and their attitude changed. Becky was pleased that they hadn't been able to tell she was mentally handicapped."

Dad wrote that Becky's psychiatrist had told him that "a few years ago he wasn't sure Becky could make it but that now he thinks she can be independent, have a job, and maybe get married one day." But Becky was afraid to think that far ahead. When her fears about the future surface, she wrote to me, "I try to decide what to do and need a little push." Making an astute observation, she says she's worried that "when I go home mom and dad will treat me like a little girl and I don't want that because I will go backward instead of forward." Yet she also longs for them to make the decision for her: "I wish mom and dad would tell me that I have to go home and that's it."

After Becky agreed to return to Honolulu to live, a new worry surfaces: Mom and Dad have suggested that she not live at home but in an apartment with a roommate. Becky wrote to me,

I feel I am still not ready to live with someone, and still not capable to make it work, and make new friends. Could you come from New York at Christmas? I am sitting here with tears in my eyes. What I really want now is to live with Mom and Dad and show them I have

*grow up a lot. But they want me to live with a roommate. Please help
me out.*

A week later she had come to terms with the new plan and writes
with a sense of pride, "I get to live like you do in apartment with
someone. I have prayed for it and dream about what it would be like. I
need a paid job and a roommate who understand me. I am a lot
different than you or anyone else in our family, cause I need extra help
and caring." I was then living in New York City with a roommate who
taught cello at the nearby Manhattan School of Music. I wrote Becky
that I liked coming home from work to hear her playing the cello, as it
reminded me of our father. I added that having a roommate always
means having problems, but that you can work them out.

ASSESSMENT

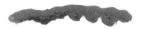

AFTER BECKY RETURNED TO HONOLULU, she underwent a number of tests to assess her cognitive abilities. Mom wrote to me, "On a test of visual memory, where they show you a triangle for a few seconds and then ask you to reproduce it, Becky couldn't do it. When she did attempt to draw some shapes, they looked as though they had been made by a child."

No one was surprised that Becky's worst results came in the area of quantitative reasoning. Mom commented that she was assessed at "about Grade 4 here. And reading is higher, 6th or low 7th grade level." But in abstract reasoning Becky rated above the mean. This astonished the psychologist, who wondered how Becky could take abstract ideas and use logic to bring them to the right conclusion, and still do so poorly on math. When Mom told me, I laughed and said that I'd been getting away with this for years.

With the help of a social worker, Becky obtained a volunteer job as a teacher's aide at a school for the blind. She liked working there but it was difficult for her to stick to a routine. As an incentive, Mom and Dad decided to pay her the minimum wage every day she went to work. Mom wrote, "I think it's working. She was down to almost nothing in her bank account and can see that her income is in direct proportion to her going to work."

The testing pointed to the complex and contradictory nature of Becky's condition and the difficulty that others had in trying to help her. As Mom wrote, "One day we underestimate her potential, and the next we overestimate." That statement would ring true for anyone who knew Becky.

"I AM TRYING TO PLAY IT COOL"

AFTER RETIRING FROM THE NAVY, Dad pursued a degree at the University of Hawaii that would certify him to teach special education classes, which he did for many years. Some of his fellow students began taking Becky to movies and the beach, and Mom and Dad hoped to find a suitable roommate among them.

Becky enjoyed interviewing potential roommates and felt it was important to know if they had any hobbies, but in one letter she expresses surprise, writing, "They have more problems than I do!" Becky's first roommate was low-key and soft-spoken, and Mom and Dad hoped she would balance Becky's more volatile personality. The relationship worked well until the woman's university class schedule and a desire to spend more time with her boyfriend made Becky feel unwelcome in her own home.

Becky would take to affection like a puppy but was put off by her roommate's extreme reserve, and their relationship became not only untenable but ridiculous. Becky attempted to engage in girl talk, but as her sense of boundaries was spotty, the conversations often went awry. She had asked her roommate if she'd ever had sexual intercourse. The guarded reply she received—"I don't recall"—had baffled Becky, and in relating the story to me, she wrote, "Gee, I think you'd be able to remember something like that."

Becky's next roommates were a young couple: the woman was a PhD candidate in clinical psychology and her husband was obtaining a master's in public health. My mother wrote, "They really care, and Becky is much easier to get along with." This couple was well-situated to observe Becky's behavior with men and caution our parents about her vulnerability and increasing recklessness. But Becky was adept at deception; I may have learned from Becky's letters more about her troubled relationships with men than her roommates or our parents.

Becky wrote that "a cute guy lives next door, and I hear someone say he wants to do the chasing on me. Well I just want him as a friend and that's it. Now I am trying to play it cool and when I see him I can just say hi and that's it. It hard to play it cool, when you live right next door to someone. So I been cleaning my apartment and I arrange the furniture around."

My heart sank, as I knew that Becky's idea of "playing it cool" meant that she'd already begun to obsess about this man, and I wasn't surprised that a few months later Becky wrote to me: "I am in love with him because he is taller than me and good-looking. How I feel about him I can't explain at all. I know I am hard to get to know. Some people never understand me. When I tell them I am a slow learner they turn away. But he didn't do that. He likes my new hair cut. It's a shag. It's easy to take care of and it shapes my face really well." Predictably, this relationship did not last.

But it meant a great deal to Becky to have a boyfriend. She wrote,

I daydream an awful lot like I picture how things will be better for me like when a boy asks me to go out with him, and after a while we are going together and his friends are jealous of me. Also he will say I am cute and hopes I am not going with anybody. But I been doing an awful lot of thinking about me—no matter how such I change myself I still do a lot of my old ways.

When Becky became involved with another neighbor, her letters express less fantasy and more anguish. She had chased after this man but became discouraged when they met only for sex. After he dumped her, Becky wrote, "OK, it was bound to happen. I asked him if we still be friends. At least he said he likes me, but that's not much to go on." She couldn't resist having sex with him in his apartment one afternoon, but that night he went out with a new girlfriend. Becky wrote, "I saw them holding hands and cried."

Becky wrote once more about the man, "I'm trying to move on, but it's hard because he still lives in the building." She added, "It's hard to forget a person who you had sex with." She writes that she's stopped calling or writing the man and has tossed out things that reminded her of him. "I am talking less about him, too, " she writes, adding, "I've decided to grow my hair down to my shoulders, and live one day at a time."

As I had cautioned her not to get involved with this man, she asked, "How did you know he was using me? I cannot seem to figure it out at all." She added, "I came to a decision to write to you since we alike in a lot of ways. I'll admit this to you but please don't tell mom & dad, that I feel guilty cause I knew he was taking advantage of me, but . . . that's the hard part. I took advantage of him for the pleasure of sex."

I recognized Becky's guilt, as I had finally come to acknowledge the way I had used my first sexual partner, subconsciously choosing a married man because I was afraid of a relationship that required true commitment. I reminded Becky that she had scolded me about that affair, and that she had been right. I was then living in New York City, having my own troubles after a series of short-lived relationships with men. I answered every one of Becky's letters but felt helpless to offer anything but general advice. I shared my concerns about her with our parents, and Mom reported that Becky had expressed appreciation for the way I was trying to help her. Mom wrote, "She said that 'because Kathy and I are so much alike she can put my thoughts into words.' How do you like that?"

When I met David, the man who would become my husband, Becky told me she was jealous. But once she met David and realized how much he liked her, she began consulting him about her problems with men, writing: "I am confused about what it means to have a heavy relationship between women and men. It's hard to even talk to guys as a friend. So what am I going to do? You can help me out about it. I will not get my hopes up too high." One of my Bennington mentors, the poet Ben Belitt, used to say that "our words are wiser than we are." I think of that when I read Becky's letters. On the surface they're a confusing jumble, but an undercurrent carries a tangle of emotions; her words reveal far more than Becky realizes. Fantasizing and hoping unrealistically was what Becky always did in a relationship, and at some level she realized it enough to express it in writing.

Becky reports that loneliness weighs on her: "I know I got to widen my interests and communicate with people. Can you give me ideas that most young people enjoy doing? I feel like an old maid." She was twenty-two.

"THEY TRY TO GET
ME DRUNK"

BECKY'S DESPERATE SEARCH for male companionship sometimes put her in danger, and she narrowly escaped being gang-raped by
some young men she met in a bar. "They try to get me drunk," she
wrote, "but I got out." When she told her roommates about the incident they informed our parents, which Becky had been afraid to do.
She wrote to me that her roommates "help me get myself back together
mentally, but it hard when you nearly been raped. It can scare you a hell
of a lot and even when you try to go forward it's hard to do after something like this."

Becky began to have nightmares and told her roommates that she
was scared to go out on her own. As painful memories of the
molestation that had occurred on the *Lurline* resurfaced, Becky's
roommates were well-equipped to listen and help. They supported
Becky when she enrolled in a job placement program, taking classes
on how to dress for interviews and how to fill out application forms.
But discouragement was lurking. With a typical mix of realism and
absurdity Becky wrote to me, "I can't be a secretary because I can't
type. I don't want to be a go-go dancer or have to work with money."

Becky felt guilty for continuing to think about her neighbor and
confessed that she was still writing him letters about how his rejection
made her feel. "I realize I was chasing him," she wrote, adding, "I
decide to keep busy more and not write or speak to him at all." But she

can't resist writing him one final letter. "It was a really bitchy letter," she wrote to me, "I did it to try to get him out of my mind."

David and I encouraged her to keep writing in a journal as a way of baring her innermost thoughts. Most writers do this, we told her, adding that it's often best to resist the impulse to share those thoughts with others.

When Becky became involved with another young man, she described him in a letter as "nice, he respect me for myself and if I don't want sex it's cool." But he was using marijuana and wanted Becky to take LSD with him, which she had the good sense to refuse. She explained to me that she said no because "I feel that everyone will make fun of me. It has happened to me before." She became disillusioned when the man took advantage of Becky's willingness to loan him money until her checking account was nearly empty.

When Becky discussed this boyfriend with her psychiatrist, he advised her to get rid of him. He also warned our parents about the man, and Dad asked Becky's roommates to tell him if the boyfriend ever came to their apartment. My mother wrote me that when he did come looking for Becky, "the roommates confronted him and told him, 'You be kind to her, no drugs, no messing with her mind.' And they supervised the visit." Mom commented, "I don't think he's a bad kid, just dumb. But he hasn't always been honest. We all agree that Becky's been going backwards, and he has not helped her." She asked me to write to Becky about this, and I did. Becky replied that she was grateful for the help she'd received in getting this man out of her life, but she still wanted a boyfriend.

THE MARY OF
EGYPT CONNECTION

BY MY MIDTWENTIES I was ready to commit to a marriage. But Becky's devastating lack of judgment when it came to men continued into her thirties. My parents' letters and phone calls became full of anxiety over Becky's reckless sexual behavior. I had thought of her as having a strong but normal libido for a young woman but at the time didn't understand that a psychiatrist would label her behavior as clinically hypersexual.

As with so many other aspects of Becky's life, I have to ask, What is normal? Many women pursue men who treat them badly and spurn those who care for them. When I met the man who would become my husband, I was in my late twenties, and it was my first experience of affection with no agenda, no hint of emotional manipulation or abuse. Like Becky I'd been slow to let go of a fantasy that had prevented me from giving or receiving genuine love.

The story of Mary of Egypt intrigued me when I first heard it years ago, but only recently have I come to understand that this is partly because of the way it connects with Becky. Venerated in the Eastern Orthodox and Coptic churches but less known in the West, Mary, a young woman living in the port city of Alexandria, was known to be sexually voracious. Joining a group of pilgrims sailing to Jerusalem, she seduced a number of men on the ship.

In Jerusalem, when Mary arrived at the door of the Church of the Holy Sepulchre, an invisible force prevented her from entering.

Weeping, she prayed to Mary the Mother of God to help her, and after entering the church and venerating the cross, she went into the desert where she lived as a hermit for many years.

A monk discovered her there when she was an old woman, so ferocious looking that at first he thought she was a wild beast. Overcoming his fear, he approached her and soon discovered that although Mary had never received any religious instruction, she knew of Jesus and the Holy Spirit and could cite Scripture passages. Recognizing God's hand in Mary's life, he asked her to pray for him.

This is one of many ancient stories of monks humbled by women, even notoriously sinful women, when they were made to realize that a lifetime of dutiful daily prayer and study might count for little compared to the life of someone who had received unwarranted grace directly from God.

My sister received conventional religious instruction as a child, but I believe it mostly seemed abstract and remote. Becky liked the song "Jesus Loves Me," its words providing her with a basic sense of security. It was many years later that I discovered that Becky harbored within a secret sense of God, and especially Jesus, as being active in her life.

"I AM HAVING PROBLEMS SEEING EYE TO EYE WITH MEN"

THE WORK AVAILABLE TO BECKY was repetitive and boring, and relationships with men provided the drama she craved. She said of a man she met at a sheltered workshop,

> We get along pretty good. I don't want to be too tied down with him. But something tells me he want the heavy relationship with me, I am going to ask for advice on what style of clothes look good on me. Also would I look good in long hair? How can I tell if men are really interested in me as a human being and not some body for sex then leave me. I am having problems seeing eye to eye with men on this subject. How in the world am I going to keep my feelings under control about love?

She says this man has told her that he

> wants a relationship with no boundaries. But I am not sure what he means. If you be a slow learner and you want to tell him about it how would you do it? This is why I feel he won't understand about it. Shit, I don't want anybody taking advantage of me just because I am slow. Like I been hurt so many times before, I just won't put up with that any more. I can't understand why he isn't coming over like he used to. Lately I been making the moves. Someone who was interested in you,

would they come over more to see you? Also I been trying to get my
skin cleared up but lately my face been going bad again with pimples.
Take care of yourself. Boy I am sure going weird.

Love, Becky.

These letters encapsulate the mood swings that were to cause Becky much trouble later in her life. After this relationship ended in disappointment she wrote, "I am frustrated with myself. I went through my old clothes. Getting rid of things helps for a while, but then I start feeling sad again." She adds, "I been doing some serious thinking how I can change myself for the better." Not long after that she wrote, "You not going to believe this, but I have changed. I avoid bad guys and enjoy life more, and when I'm in a depressed mood I been talking more to people about it and it helps. Also I try to look nicer when I go to work. I'm lucky to have a job that I enjoy." But this job, like most of them, did not last. When a coworker yelled at her she quit, staying home and moping.

"IT SEEMS LIKE I DON'T LIKE THE MEN WHO LIKE ME"

I HAD MET MY FUTURE HUSBAND in New York City, and in 1974 we moved to my mother's hometown in western South Dakota. Her parents had died, and Mom needed time to decide what to do with the house in which she had been raised, and the farm and ranch land she'd inherited. It seemed an appropriate move for us at the time; we felt that the quiet of a small, remote town would be good for our writing.

Becky wrote me letters nearly every day. She liked the idea of me and David living in our grandparents' house and shared some memories of being there as a child. She also wrote about the men in her life with a dizzy momentum, rushing from "How can I tell when a guy is using me for my body?" to "I bought a new pants suit at the thrift store because its color brings out my eyes."

One major theme is her suspicion that the men she was infatuated with might not respect her, combined with her desire to be attractive to men. I tried to tell her that she was expressing openly what many women feel but try to keep hidden. We want to be attractive because we know that men judge us on our appearance, but we also want a man who loves and respects us for who we are.

Former boyfriends continue to be a problem. One makes prank calls, another gives her phone number to friends. Becky writes that she received a phone call from a stranger, and says that "I feel it was someone looking for an easy lay." Mom and Dad are forced to change their number. After Becky meets one young man through a mutual friend, she writes to me that "mom thinks he's boring." But Becky is beginning to think that boring is good. "He took me out and didn't make a pass at me," she writes. "He is treating me like a lady." But like her other relationships, this one doesn't last. She writes, "It seems like I don't like the men who like me. I like the other kind, but am trying to like the nice men now." She remains unconvinced when I try to tell her that I have faced the same problem, one that many women face: being attracted to men who are wrong for us and being slow to appreciate a man who appreciates us.

Becky's obsession with men lasted well past adolescence, and my mother, ever the realist, began to discuss with Becky the possibility of becoming sterilized so that she would not risk becoming pregnant. Dad was reluctant, still hoping that Becky could one day have a family. But Becky decided to have the procedure. She liked children but had come to realize that even with family support she wasn't capable of raising a child.

I used to wonder if Becky would ever grow beyond the emotional age of fourteen. For years, she would ask me to buy specific brands of shampoo, sunscreen, or toothpaste. When I asked her why, she explained that she'd seen the products advertised on television. Becky was exactly the audience marketers have in mind, a gullible girl with a low IQ who readily engages in magical thinking: *If I use this toothpaste or drink this soda, I'll be with people doing fun things together. I will attract a handsome guy.*

One year Becky asked my parents for a "glamour shot" session with a photographer. Our sister Charlotte had done this and Becky liked the results, but she was afraid to go on her own. She wanted me to take her and get a glamour shot as well. I'd rather spend an hour in the dentist's chair than endure a makeup session, but I had to say yes.

Becky received the ministrations of the cosmetician with a solemn air, as if she were in church receiving Communion. Her sallow skin, marked with pocks and deep worry lines, became smooth under foundation makeup and contoured blush. As her face transformed before her eyes, Becky became quiet, no longer joking about how jealous her friends would be to see her now.

The revelation for all of us that day—Becky, me, the genial photographer, and the makeup artist—was how easy it was to make Becky over. She'd been blessed with the natural curl of our father's hair, and just a few minutes in hot rollers gave her big hair, which delighted her. Awestruck, she said, "I look like I belong on TV."

I came out of the experience looking much like myself, if a bit more polished. Becky came out looking like a different person. And that was the point. From the time she was a teenager, Becky had longed for what she considered a normal life, one that included romance and marriage. Now, as a pretty woman emerged, one who could attract a man, she said, "Look at me. Just look at me." It sounded like a prayer.

PART THREE

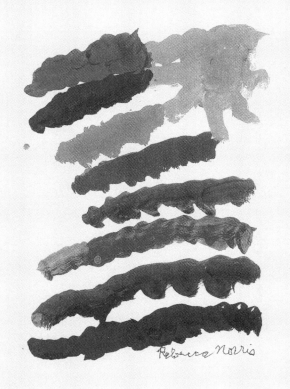

Rebecca Norris

"What Can I Do to Be Good Enough to Develop Skills?"

"A BIG POODLE IN THE DOG HOUSE"

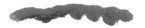

Becky's roommates informed Mom and Dad that once they obtained their degrees they'd be leaving for the US mainland. They also warned Mom and Dad that Becky was not handling even her limited independence well. A social worker suggested that Becky move into a group home, but her psychiatrist thought that she might be better off living with her family again. So Becky moved back home with Mom, Dad, and Charlotte.

Employment remained a concern. Because of her experience caring for disabled children at Devereux, Becky hoped to become a caregiver or nursing aide but had to settle for working as a restaurant dishwasher. She found that job too physically taxing and, true to form, began missing days until she was fired. But not working meant that her funds were low again. She wrote, "Now I got to budget better. But I couldn't say no to an Avon lady—I bought $30.00 worth of things, then had to call to tell her I couldn't afford it. I need to learn to say no to people."

Becky's love of gossip and a penchant for meddling in the affairs of others continued to be a problem for her at work. After she was fired from yet another job, our parents arranged for her to do daily chores around the house in exchange for pay. Becky writes, "I feel like a big poodle in the dog house. When I don't have a job I get the cold shoulder at home."

With a flash of self-awareness Becky wrote, "I know I am playing games with myself. I try to be an adult now." When she learns that a nearby YMCA is hiring "special" people for their new restaurant called the Breadline, she applies for a job on her own. "But," she writes to me, "most days I lie on my back and want to give up on life. I am having an awful time struggling for independence. I know in time I'll be able to live a normal life like everyone. I feel frustrated in my life . . . Kathy did you ever feel like this when you're growing up?" I responded by saying that I knew how scary independence could be, but I was proud of her for being willing to try a new kind of job.

When Becky was hired at the Breadline, she told me she was looking forward to working there. But before her first day there, without telling anyone, she sent the café manager a letter turning down the job. Dad managed to straighten things out, and this became Becky's most long-lasting and best experience of work.

"I TRY TO CHANGE
FOR A NEW ME"

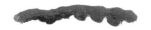

BECKY'S FIRST JOB AT the Breadline was answering the phone. Then she bussed tables. She wrote, "I scared to do it but I feel it's better to get as many experiences as I can." She was thrilled when coworkers invited her to join them for pizza after work. The Breadline paid for her to receive speech therapy at the University of Hawaii across the street from the restaurant, and this boosted her confidence when she began to work as a hostess. Mom took friends to the restaurant one day for lunch and reported that Becky "seemed quite professional and obviously took pride in her appearance."

But in her letters to me Becky continued to reveal her anxieties. "I like the people at Breadline but can't take the pressure in restaurant work. How do you do a new self-image? Maybe I'm setting my goal too high for me and that's why it doesn't work out."

When Becky started not showing up for work or calling in sick, she wrote, "I really unhappy with myself for doing the same thing over and over. People talk to me about it but I'm the one who's got to take some action." I tried to convince her that she was not alone in this, that everyone contends with bad habits they want to change. She said of herself, "I whine too much, I complain when I'm sick, and don't answer the phone or door when I don't feel like it," and seemed surprised to hear that sometimes I struggled with these things as well. She couldn't resist admonishing me: "Write more to me and less to parents," and chided me severely when I failed to send her a Valentine. "I was expecting a soupy card from you and when it didn't come it hurt my feelings awful bad."

Becky often wrote letters to express her frustrations rather than confront people in person. My parents found this note one day on the kitchen table:

Mom and Dad,

I scared to grow up and except responsibles on my own. I not very reliable. It hard for me to take pressure, when I let little things upset me, and I don't show up to work. I was fine Monday but working as a waitress I get all freak out. So I went Tuesday even when I didn't feel like it. I try to change for a new me. I try to hold down a job but I don't control my feelings very good. I don't want to be on Welfare. I bought a math book to improve my skills so when I buy something I will know when I get the right change. I think I did right by getting a math book. But today I did wrong by not going to work or calling ahead of time. I am not pretty at all when I am negative all the time. It's hard living with you, you make me uptight when I try my best to do things around the house I get a lecture every time, or when I do good by going to work you don't discuss how my day was and interrupt me when I do talk about it.

Becky

The Breadline staff convinced her to stick with the job, and when their attempts to train her as a cashier failed, they enrolled Becky in a math class at a community college. But Becky writes that her life is "a mess, and I probably make it this way." She asks me, "Did you ever have these struggles, when you didn't want your parents to help out, and you wanted to make your own plans for the future?" She adds, "I know mom and dad don't want to see me hurt, but how can I live my life if they don't let go of this little bird who wants to make it in this world?"

One significant change that's disturbing Becky is that our brother, John, and his wife, Marilyn, have moved to Hawaii with their infant daughter, and the plan is for our parents to sell their current home and buy a larger one that can accommodate everyone. Until a new house is found, the family is crammed into the old one, and one day when Becky was in a foul mood, her yelling and slamming doors woke the baby from a nap. "Everyone got after me," she complains, "and I felt sorry about the baby, but she got back to sleep."

Once the family moves, Becky likes having her own room for the privacy it affords. But when the Breadline had to let her go because of her erratic behavior, she became depressed. Becky was only occasionally attending church with Mom and Dad, but her belief that angels were active in our lives remained strong. This letter reached me in South Dakota:

To Kathy,

As I woke up to get myself breakfast I saw a beautiful sunrise. It beautiful than used to my image picture. I saw your lovely face in the clouds. Could be I was think about you and David wishing it would be beautiful for you in every way and happiness too. Angels guarding you and they a different color than the clouds. I am thank for to be able to see with my two eyes being able to see what I want to see.

Love Becky

THE FINDER OF LOST THINGS

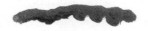

IT MADE SENSE FOR THE FAMILY to pool resources and purchase a home that was large enough for everyone in the family. The house they found in Mānoa Valley, a residential neighborhood of Honolulu, was on a lot with many fruit trees and flowered hedges, and the front lanai had a large porch swing that was put to good use. The main floor included a library that served as a nursery for the children who lived in the house over the twenty years my family was there. Eventually there were four: John and Marilyn's two daughters and Charlotte's daughter and son.

Every evening the family exercised triage along the steep driveway, parking cars according to who had to leave first in the morning. Marilyn left around 5 a.m. for her job as a financial planner. Mom was next, leaving for her long commute to teach at an elementary school in Pearl City. Then Charlotte drove downtown to her job at a law firm. As a United Church of Christ pastor, my brother had a more flexible schedule, as did my father, who worked nights as a musician. One of them drove the children to school. When one niece was in kindergarten and a teacher asked her when was a good time to call to speak to someone in her family, she replied, "You can call anytime. Someone's always there."

The living arrangement gave the children in the household a considerable sense of security. And somehow it worked. Becky helped with the laundry, picked things up around the house, and performed a number of kitchen duties. On most nights the family ate together, but the conversations of our intensely verbal family could leave Becky feeling excluded. She was capable of comprehending more than most people gave her credit for, but at times we went too fast for her. If she complained, we'd slow down a bit and make more of an effort to include her. But it could be difficult, as Becky expressed little interest in the work that others in the family were doing. She occasionally asked John what he'd be preaching on, but I can't recall her ever asking me about what I was reading or writing.

Our nephew, the youngest member of the household, says that Becky was often the only person who would play with him. They'd sit on the floor and play board games for hours, and when he donned an old Halloween costume to act out a fantasy, Becky was his avid audience. When he thought Becky wasn't getting the respect she deserved, he spoke up. One night at dinner my dad was scolding Becky, and he told his grandfather to back off. He was only five years old, but his outburst stopped my dad. "I could tell he felt bad about what he'd been saying," he says, adding that "after that Auntie B would take me aside and say, 'You stuck up for me and I'll stick up for you.'"

My parents offered some child care, as did Becky, who became known as the Finder of Lost Things, a useful skill in a large household with young children. One morning Marilyn became frantic when she was fixing breakfast for her girls and lost a contact lens. She didn't have a replacement and needed to drive the girls to swimming lessons. Becky opened the refrigerator door, which my sister-in-law had recently opened to get milk, and immediately spied the lens near the butter dish.

Our family has plenty of stories like this. Becky could find "lost" people as well; she outdid all of us at remembering names, even those of people we hadn't seen in years. The brain is a mystery, and I believe my sister's brain was even more mysterious than most. Her ability to find lost objects and name lost people can't be explained. Becky attributed it to her guardian angel helping her out.

Becky's increasing instability—she was later diagnosed as having bipolar disorder—was becoming more pronounced, and my dad noted that "Becky's problems become our problems." When she was on a high she became a "a tornado of energy," writing dozens of letters to friends and family. He drily noted that of all of the family members, "she's the one who is most in touch with her feelings—and she shares them with us all."

But Becky was still stable enough to be trusted to pick up her two oldest nieces from their nearby elementary school and bring them home. One recalls that she was always happy when Becky showed up, as she walked more slowly than the other adults in the family and often stopped at a neighborhood park where she and her sister could play. Another remembers that Becky would sometimes take them to an ice cream parlor, a secret they kept from her parents. The girls have fond memories of these afternoons, and Becky was proud to be their caregiver. When she won a five-hundred-dollar shopping spree at a weekly contest run by a local paper, the article quotes her as saying, "Wow, I won. This is the first time I've ever won anything." When asked by the reporter where she worked, she replied that she looked after her nieces and a nephew. Becky kept the clipping in a small box with family photos and other precious possessions.

"I WANT TO CHANGE BUT AM AFRAID OF CHANGE"

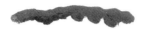

MY HUSBAND DAVID AND I were usually able to come to Hawaii in December and stay with my family over the Christmas holidays. David enjoyed the unaccustomed opportunity to cook for more than the two of us, and the children looked forward to the chocolate mousse he made from scratch and the omelets I prepared for them on request. They nicknamed David "Uncle Mousse." I was "Auntie Omelet."

Becky, Charlotte, and I enjoyed festooning the tree every year with decorations that had been in the family since we were children. The house had a fireplace with a mantel that was perfect for hanging five homemade stockings, one for each child and one for Becky. Early on Christmas morning, Becky would join the children on the second floor before descending stairs to find out what Santa had brought. We knew that Becky would soon become exhausted and weepy and need some time to herself, and later in the day we'd have to coax her into posing for an annual family photo.

I learned that even when I was present, Becky often preferred to communicate in writing and would place long notes in her loopy handwriting on my pillow or in a book I was reading. One that I received the day after she'd been arguing with our parents and cross with me began:

Kathy,

I want to go out with you later today, just the two of us. Just want to think things out. I can tell you something that's been bugging me but I can't do anything about it. I am really scared to be sufficient on my own. I always will be dependent on other people. I want to change but am afraid of change. I know I did wrong yesterday but Dad and Mom keep bringing up situations after they're dead. I am not ready to be married but there's a lot of things I want to change. I have a child side that I need to work on. It's hard to change things on my own. I always get into situations and can't do the adult thing. I get this way a lot. I sorry I yell at you. I want to be more dependable on my own but I don't understand how to be a woman. It always seem I grew up too fast and I'd like to discuss this with you. This has to be confidential between us.

Writing letters was how Becky dealt with the basic questions of life, and her reference to growing up too fast was a sure sign that the sex abuse she'd experienced at thirteen still haunted her. But what was urgent in one moment would become insignificant in the next. It was difficult to respond, and I knew that the next time I saw her she would be less likely to talk about her fears than to ask me to take her shopping.

"I FEEL LOST AGAIN"

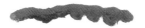

AS BECKY ENTERED HER LATE TWENTIES, the consequences of her being "borderline" became more evident. She grew bored with repetitive tasks, but when she was placed in a regular work environment, she couldn't handle the demands placed on her. Yet she persisted, enrolling in one job training program after another.

After yet another program she'd enrolled in ended, she wrote to me, "I feel lost again and depressed. This happens every time, and I'm back to square one." When Becky tells a social worker that she feels overprotected living at home, the woman asks if she's ever considered living in a group home. She arranges for Becky to spend a night in a place that has an opening, and Becky writes to me that "it went very well. I felt at home there." But she learns that she won't qualify for a group home until she has Social Security disability income. Mom and Dad were willing to do the required paperwork but were still reluctant to admit that Becky might be better off living apart from the family.

Their letters to me reveal their sense of impending crisis, as Becky was beginning to show signs of the hypersexuality that is a symptom of bipolar disorder. Lately their main concern, Dad wrote, was that Becky had been "trying to put the make on every workman who comes to the house." He became angry when he discovered that Becky had lied about canceling an appointment with a tutor and spent the afternoon instead with the men who had installed solar panels on the roof. Becky was aware of doing wrong but unable to control herself.

With typical insight she wrote to me, "I start to see a pattern in my life and I would like to change it."

When some odd-looking mail arrived at the house addressed to Becky, Dad discovered that she'd been answering lonely hearts advertisements. He intercepted one letter and pointed out to Becky that it was obscene and the man was obviously sick. Becky knew she'd made a stupid mistake but said that she wanted male friends.

One November Becky scolded me and my husband for failing to send her a birthday card in October: "You skipped a very important day." She told us that she's been feeling down but has been walking for exercise and is wearing bright lipstick to cheer herself up. She includes in her letter a typically specific list of the things she wants for Christmas: "make-up lessons; lipsticks in red, pink, and plum; knee-high socks in crazy patterns; a nightgown with long sleeves; word-seek puzzles; books; crayons; drawing paper."

Becky also writes that she met a man at a bus stop and gave him her name and address. "I had Charlie cologne on, nice make-up, and a new hair cut. I've been going for a new image, and I think it worked on him." She was impressed that he didn't put her down after she told him about being in a program for people with learning difficulties. Becky writes to me, "I made the first move, and left a note for him at work. He said he'd call but didn't." She asks, plaintively, "How do you just let things happen without pushing too hard?" She also writes to my husband separately for advice: "I want to know," she asks, "what do men want in a woman? Is playing hard to get good for their ego?"

As another birthday approached, Becky writes to my husband, "I not sure you want another depressed letter from me. But I need advice. I met a guy on the bus and we went to his place and had sex. And then Dad was upset because he came up to the house. I'm confused. Do guys want sex more than women, and do they drop you afterward?"

Dad tells me that when a stranger phoned asking for Becky, she said she didn't want to talk to him. After Dad relayed the message the man said, "Well she asked me to call her; we're supposed to have a date tonight." Becky yelled, "I told him I'm not going out with him because he's married!" He adds, "It was loud enough for him to hear, and he hung up. I talked with her about how she gets herself into these situations but expects us to help her get out of them. What a mess. I try to assume the survival technique your mother has learned with regard to Becky: stoicism."

NOT STOICISM
BUT STABILITY

STOICISM ISN'T EXACTLY THE RIGHT WORD to describe my mother's attitude toward Becky or to life itself. Like her mother, she had a stability that I believe was grounded in a rock-solid Christian faith. But neither of them spoke much about it. The Norris side of my family was much more volatile. My Grandfather Norris was saved at a tent revival meeting in the early twentieth century, worked his way through West Virginia Wesleyan, and served as a pastor for the rest of his life. He married the young woman who'd been playing piano at the revival; her Christianity was fervent and vocal.

I've long been grateful that my family heritage contains two distinct versions of the Christian faith. My appreciation of that may be one reason I was attracted to the Benedictines, who make vows that are unique to their order—to remain stable but also open to change.

Becky and I spent much more time with our Grandmother Totten than our Grandmother Norris, and I believe that her quiet trust in God was formative for both of us. It provided us with hope and an unshakable confidence that made us more ready to accept and endure whatever came our way.

"ALL MY DREAMS GET SUNK"

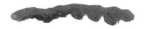

WHEN BECKY'S DOCTOR CONVINCES her of the dangers of mixing alcohol with psychotropic medications, she begins attending AA meetings. She tells me she likes her sponsor, an older woman who asks Becky to call her *tutu*, the Hawaiian word for "grandmother." "She said she's there for me any time," adding that "this is helpful since I'm new at this and feeling scared."

After a few months Becky begins to skip meetings and makes so many demands of her sponsor that the woman asks her not to call any more. She's also canceling appointments with her psychiatrist. She writes to me that "it seems that lately I been changing but for the worst. It's really hard for me to grow up and I don't know how. I'm 31 years old, no friends, no job, overweight. I don't exercise and turn down invitations to go out." She enjoyed a picnic at a beach park with my brother, his wife, and their two young daughters. But this is an increasingly rare bright spot in her life.

Dad has high hopes for a new psychiatrist. But Becky confides that she is "really worried about my life. Without my loving and caring family, I won't survive. But all my dreams get sunk, and I lie in bed and cry and can't sleep."

During a long walk with me at Christmas, Becky broods on the past, the childhood molestation, the gang assault she had narrowly avoided, and her many bad relationships with men. I'm convinced that given Becky's eagerness to please others, many of her sexual experiences amounted to rape. The next day Becky leaves me a note: "It is hard growing up, when I had a lot of bad experiences in my childhood and I get flashbacks. Sometimes they wake me up and I worry so much I can't sleep at night." Then, as usual, she abruptly changes the subject: "I'd like to know how to wear different tops and pants and what colors look good on me."

The next year when I phone on her birthday, she won't talk to me. Later she writes to explain that she was in a bad mood that day and offers to let us have her room when David and I return for Christmas. She enrolls in an exercise class at a YMCA, but her enthusiasm wanes when the instructor scolds her about not trying hard enough. She writes to me that she replied, "I'm doing the best I can," and quits the class.

"My fears are getting bigger," she writes, adding, "I don't know what I want in life. Been watching TV and that's it. Scared of living and dying. Do you know how long to keep eye make-up? I read it's best to throw it out after three months." Mom and Dad were pleased that when they made a trip to Europe, Becky did well in their absence, helping take care of the house and our brother's young girls. But a crisis was brewing.

PART FOUR

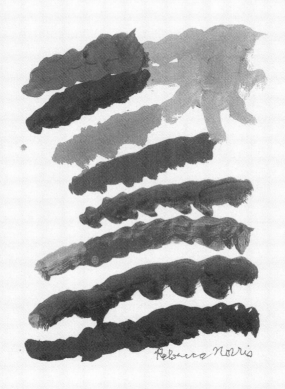

Rebecca Norris

*"What Does 'Being
Dependent' Mean?"*

"I KNOW GOD HAS A PLAN FOR ME"

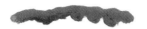

BECKY WROTE TO ME that new medication is making her hyper, and she's keeping others in the family awake at night. She frequently wets her bed. Writing letters to me and David apparently provides some relief. "In a way you're my doctor," she writes, "so I can write my troubles and forget them." She reports that when an old boyfriend took her to a movie, she snuck out and walked home without saying goodbye. "Every time I do normal things I get tired out," she writes. "I know God has a plan for me and it will be all right in the future. But I worry."

Dad reports that "Becky is seeing her shrink today, something she's been refusing to do for the last few months. It's a relief," he adds, "even though the bills are high. But we've been living with unpredictable behavior and suicide threats." Becky is demonstrating little understanding of the consequences of her words and actions. Her doctor, knowing that Becky was sexually active, had warned her about AIDS, so she went to a clinic and got tested for HIV. Then she called a boyfriend's mother, and said, "I tested negative, but I'll let you know if I ever get AIDS." She was surprised and hurt when the woman became upset and told her never to contact her son again.

For the first time in her life, Becky was in trouble with the law. She had met a man who worked at a nearby shopping center and had sex with him. After he dumped her, she began stalking him, and he had her served with a restraining order. One day, when she knew he was at work, she broke into his apartment and trashed it. Dad wrote that Becky had not only wrecked the man's apartment, she told him she had AIDS. "When Becky feels scorned," he wrote, "she can be vicious." She's facing a contempt of court citation that could lead to a prison sentence, but in her letters to me she never mentions her crime and says little about the man, only that she's stopped contacting him. But it's clear that she doesn't grasp the seriousness of her situation when she writes that she is "thinking of waiting a while and then writing to apologize to him and also the police detective who came to the house. Do you think I should get a permanent? I can get a cheap one at the community college." Dad covered the man's expenses for repairs to his apartment and by the grace of God Becky received therapy instead of a prison sentence.

All of us wanted to share Becky's faith that God had a plan for her, but it was too difficult to maintain that hope. Becky was raised in a churchgoing household, but even the pastors in the family—my brother and also Marilyn, who'd become an Episcopal priest—didn't tend to discuss with family members the idea of God directing our lives. But it makes sense to me that as Becky's mental state deteriorated, she turned to her childhood faith in God, faith in a God who loved and cared for her even when she misbehaved. But we became increasingly concerned when Becky's inability to control herself became more pronounced, and her behavior became as erratic as her prose.

Becky's new recklessness came to a head one night when, as my dad wrote to me, "A man walked her home, a good-looking guy with long hair, barefoot, bare-chested and wearing shorts. When she got him to the door she left him there, ran upstairs, locked herself in her room, and took a shower. He wandered up the stairs looking for her and found your mom pedaling on her exercise bike watching the nightly news.

Then he wandered over to your brother, who was alarmed at the sight of this stranger in his kids' room. I was so busy at my computer that I missed all of this, but heard a strange voice and got up to investigate."

Dad drove the man a few blocks to the main road and then tried to convince Becky that anyone she brought home was her responsibility. The next night the man returned, drunk and looking for Becky. When he was refused entry to the house, he muttered threats and left. But he returned a few days later and when he was told that Becky wasn't home, he went into a neighbor's garage and stretched across the top of their car to sleep. As these neighbors were away on vacation, my father called the police. He wrote that this young man "appeared dangerous, but I had no idea where he lived or what his name was."

When Becky came home later that day, Dad confronted her about the danger to the entire family posed by her involvement with this stranger. She stormed out of the house and did not return that night, a Tuesday. On Wednesday my parents expected a call from her, but none came. On Thursday Dad filed a missing person report. Mom held out hope, but Dad was convinced that Becky was dead and checked at the city morgue.

My father's band, the New Orleans Jazz Band of Hawaii, was then playing from 5 p.m. to 9 p.m. six nights a week at Trappers, a nightclub in Waikiki. When he went to work on Thursday, my mother went with him to offer moral support. He wrote me that "I didn't tell anyone in the band about Becky, but when we got a request for 'Gypsy Rose' and I came to the line 'Baby, Baby won't you come home,' I broke down and cried. Then John called to say that Becky had walked in at about 8 p.m., surprised that we had been concerned. Lois came to the bandstand to tell me that Becky was home, and I cried again."

Dad kept Becky close all the next day, so relieved to have her home that he was glad to listen to her nonstop chatter. She soon stabilized, keeping appointments and taking her medication. But her psychiatrist advised Mom and Dad that Becky's living at home was contributing to her regression, and they finally agreed to find a group home for her. Dad was worried that Becky's seven-year-old niece, who was accustomed to playing with Becky every day after school, had been deeply affected by the family crisis, even though she adopted an air of nonchalance. When he tried to explain to her that the police had been at the house twice in a week because of her aunt's problems, she shrugged and said, "That's life!"

"IF I STAY WITH THE FAMILY
I'LL BE A FAILURE"

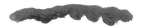

I BELIEVE MY SISTER KNEW it was time for her to leave the family nest, and some part of her wanted to go. But the thought frightened her, and unable to express this, even to herself, her mood swings became severe. My father writes that "on her down trip she sits on the couch all day and watches television. When she's up she sings loudly to the music on the radio all night."

One afternoon Becky broke a window in her room, and when Marilyn went to investigate, she found Becky sitting on the floor in a near-catatonic state. She had drunk most of a bottle of wine and hadn't noticed that her period had begun, so there was blood on her clothing and the carpet. When Marilyn called for an ambulance, Charlotte quietly shepherded the children out of the house.

As Marilyn waited with Becky in the emergency room of Tripler Army Hospital, she found that Becky seemed to be in another world, talking quietly to the hands of the clock on the wall. When a doctor brought a group of medical students to observe Becky, she asked them to leave, saying, "She's not hurting anyone. Just let her be." She remained with Becky until the sedatives she'd been given kicked in. Becky was admitted to a psychiatric hospital, Kahi Mohala, but was released after just a few days, apparently for the convenience of a doctor who was going on vacation. It was too soon: at home Becky quickly relapsed, sitting naked on the floor of her room and raving incoherently. When she returned to the hospital, Mom and Dad worried about how long they could afford to keep her there, and it was a relief when Becky's Medicaid and Social Security Disability Income were approved. It was difficult for Mom and Dad to give up their role as Becky's protectors, but they were both nearing seventy years of age and hoped that these programs would provide Becky with some security for the rest of her life.

A social worker found Becky a place in a group home; she never lived with the family again. Her psychiatrist assured our parents that they could still advocate for Becky, but she had to learn to live with other people, who would not be as indulgent as the family.

My father wrote that when this psychiatrist had taken Becky off some of her drugs she became "her old normal self, helping me prepare the jazz band's newsletter for mailing. Just a few weeks ago she was the ultimate couch potato. She would shit in her pants, and not even know it. We wondered how we were going to cope. But we are encouraged now."

Becky writes to me, "If I stay with the family I'll be a failure. I'm in tears writing this." Although she knew she needed to make this move, she found ways to rebel against it. Early one morning she ran away from the home and called Dad from a pay phone, telling him she wanted to be committed to the Hawaii State Hospital. She later wrote me, saying, "I decided that I wanted to be locked up and have all my decisions made for me." Dad agreed to drive her to the hospital. But as they neared the place Becky hesitated, asking to go to a fast-food place for breakfast. Over pancakes, she began to talk more realistically and agreed to return to the group home.

Becky's ups and downs would continue, but medication and counseling helped to keep her illness at bay. It would be over twenty years later, when Becky was approaching sixty, that another psychotic break would occur.

MRS. R.

BECKY LANDED IN A GROUP HOME with an experienced caregiver. I'll call her Mrs. R. Mom and Dad told her she could always contact them with concerns about Becky.

The relationship was not an easy one for either woman. Mrs. R. was helping Becky grow up, and Becky resisted her at every turn, slamming doors, spitting, and meddling in the affairs of other residents. Mrs. R. rolled with Becky's mood swings, telling Mom and Dad that one day Becky is yelling at her and the next day gives her the silent treatment. "She wants everything on her terms," she says, a comment that would resonate with anyone who knew Becky.

When I met Mrs. R on a Christmas visit, I was impressed by her capable and unflappable air, and her obvious concern for Becky's welfare. When I told her the story about Becky using her disability against me when we were younger, claiming that I couldn't hit her because she was retarded, she laughed. It was clear to me that Mrs. R. had a good grasp of Becky's intelligence as well as her limitations. I found it significant that although Becky constantly complained about the other women in the home, she was reticent about Mrs. R., saying only that she worked hard to take care of her and the other women. I believe Becky understood that Mrs. R. liked her and was doing her a world of good.

What none of us anticipated was that Becky would remain in this home for fifteen years, and Becky's relationship with Mrs. R. would be one of the most significant of her life.

A HAUNTING

My parents had always provided me and my siblings with a loving environment. When we faced challenges that seemed insurmountable, my mother was a source of calm, comfort, and wisdom. My father was more volatile, mixing good advice with a dose of humor or sarcasm, and getting us to laugh at ourselves.

When my father was ten, his older half brother Richard died of spinal meningitis, and Dad became the oldest child in his family, acquiring a sense of duty that endured. He looked after his younger siblings for years, and when his widowed mother was in her eighties, he rescued her from a dismal nursing home in Iowa where he found her listless, bedridden, and suffering from bedsores. After taking her to Hawaii to live with the family, he hired a physical therapist to help her learn to walk again.

There had once been a family crisis that my father had not been able to fix, and when Becky began her descent into mental illness, it must have been horrific for him to witness her decline, as his younger sister Mary had demonstrated many of the same symptoms. She had received a diagnosis of "schizophrenia, undifferentiated," and like Becky, she became sexually promiscuous. She would disappear for days, and on returning home she'd engage in frantic episodes of giving away her clothes, saying she wouldn't need them in heaven. Dad knew that Mary's promiscuity was combined with an extremely prudish attitude toward sex. She was unwilling to undress even in front of her sisters.

It was clear that Mary needed long-term treatment, but as her parents couldn't afford a private facility, she was admitted to the Independence State Hospital in Independence, Iowa. My dad was then in the US Navy Band in Washington, DC, living there with my mother and brother, a toddler, and he could rarely visit.

Doctors at the state hospital learned that when Mary was five, she had been sexually molested by her half brother Richard, who was fourteen. This occurred shortly before Richard died, and Mary told a psychiatrist that she had caused his death. She also said there was something wrong with her genitals, which had increased her sexual drive and caused her present illness. By the time she was admitted to the hospital, she'd had intercourse with a number of men and had contracted gonorrhea. And she was pregnant.

When Mary was due to give birth, she was sent to the university hospital in Iowa City; her room was considered secure as it had bars on the windows. A few days after Mary delivered a baby girl, her parents were at the hospital completing plans for the baby's adoption. Mary had wanted her child to stay in the family, but the doctors advised against it. She was scheduled to return to the state hospital where she could be given shock treatments that hadn't been possible while she was pregnant, but Mary managed to get to a room on an upper floor that had an unsecured window and jumped out.

I first learned about my Aunt Mary when I was nine years old. Looking through old photographs, I found one that was taken of my parents shortly after they were married, posing with Dad's parents and siblings in a studio that used a stained glass window as a backdrop, appropriate for a Methodist pastor and his family. I saw a woman I didn't recognize and asked Dad who she was. He sighed and told me it was his sister Mary and that she had died a few months after I was born. Over the years I learned more about Mary, but I doubt Becky knew much about her; she never mentioned her.

Mary died at twenty-six. As Becky entered her twenties my father must have been haunted as her mental illness became more pronounced. Becky's psychiatrist determined that she had bipolar disorder and not schizophrenia, and with the help of medication and counseling, Becky emerged from her crisis in relatively stable condition. But surely the memory of his sister Mary shadowed my father and contributed to his sense of guilt.

Once when Becky was depressed about losing her psychiatrist she asked Dad, "Do you know what it means to lose your best friend?" Dad didn't tell her the doctor had dropped her because he no longer took Medicaid patients. "When he gets back from his vacation," he wrote, "I'm going to call him and do a little begging."

Dad did a lot of begging on Becky's behalf. He was unsuccessful in his efforts to get the Navy to grant Becky permanent dependent status. But he made sure that Becky's physicians, counselors, and social workers knew they could consult with him at any time. He frequently listened to Mrs. R. express her frustrations in the hope that she wouldn't give up on Becky and evict her from her group home.

Dad's guilt about Becky was centered on the decision he and Mom made to use Bethesda Naval Hospital for her birth. All indications were that my sister had developed normally in the womb, and Dad felt that if they had gone to a private hospital, Mom would not have endured mistreatment and Becky would not have suffered brain damage.

While my Dad's diligence with Becky's care was admixed with a dose of guilt, I had my own burden in this regard. For many years, my connection with Becky was marked by physical distance. From the time when I went to college in 1965 to the year 2000, when my husband was diagnosed with lung cancer and we began to spend more time in Honolulu, I lived thousands of miles away from the family. I hadn't deliberately chosen to be apart from Becky for much of my life:

going to college, working in New York City, and living in South Dakota had made sense.

I'd been glad to receive Becky's many letters and responded with letters and phone calls. Becky once flew to South Dakota to stay with me and David for several weeks. But while I'd often been able to visit the family at a Christmas, I didn't live with Becky in the day to day. My sister Charlotte did, and she bore the brunt of Becky's most disturbing and destructive behavior. She also witnessed the effect it had on our parents.

Charlotte understandably felt that where Becky was concerned, she had paid her dues, and in Becky's later years as I began to take on more duties in caring for her, I knew I couldn't call on Charlotte except in an emergency. As for myself, I sometimes felt that I was attempting to make up for all the times I hadn't been there for Becky. This made it easier for me to enjoy her company, even when that meant spending an entire day with her when she was hospitalized.

Dad had taught me a lot about being indefatigable where Becky was concerned, and this was a great help when I became her advocate. Experience with my husband had taught me that every hospital patient needs someone who will stand up for them, someone willing to be there early in the morning when a doctor makes rounds and to be present at the shift changes of the the nursing staff. And Becky required extra diligence: if a doctor or nurse addressed me rather than Becky, I'd defer to her. I explained that while my sister had been brain damaged at birth, she understood a great deal about her medical history and could speak for herself.

"BECKY SAYS YOU'RE GETTING A DIVORCE"

THAT VISIT TO ME AND DAVID in South Dakota taught me that while Becky could be smart about many things, she was remarkably naive when it came to human relationships. When she witnessed one of our marital spats, with us shouting at each other until my husband left, slamming the front door behind him, Becky began to weep. I reminded her that neither David nor I had said anything cruel or mean, and I tried to reassured her that neither of us would stay angry for long, especially as we'd been fighting over something trivial—the kitchen garbage can. Becky nodded but looked doubtful.

A few days later when I was on the phone with Mom she said, "Becky says you're getting a divorce." I was startled, but when I explained what had happened Mom laughed. "It must have been serious," she said, "if it was about the kitchen garbage can."

Romantic relationships mattered to Becky, and she greatly admired couples who had weathered many decades together. Our parents were married for sixty-four years; my husband and I had thirty-one years together before he died. A man at church told me he appreciated Becky's acceptance of him and his partner. They'd been a couple for sixty years, but their families had refused to acknowledge the relationship. I was glad when he told me how much Becky's acceptance meant to him; it indicated that despite her many unfortunate experiences, Becky never lost her belief in the power of love to endure all things. But she was slow to recognize that love was more than romance and that it required daily diligence, and sometimes a silly shouting match.

In her relationships with people outside the family, Becky had experienced little of a normal, daily give and take. Thus for her, life with roommates meant doing constant battle. Even a minor dispute could escalate into a long-lasting feud. The challenges of living in a group home would prove to be a great test for both Becky and her caregivers.

"PLEASE DON'T ASK ME ABOUT MY GROUP HOME"

NOT LONG AFTER MOVING into Mrs. R.'s group home, Becky wrote to me: "I love my new place. My new doctor is nice. I'm taking lithium now and it's working OK. I also started in a new day program called the Clubhouse. I'm excited about all these positive changes." She tells me, "I can't remember much about the hospital, but a nurse told me I was taking my clothes off and yelling. This year will be better, and I won't go back to the mental hospital. How are you two doing? Have a good Easter. You are both in my prayers."

Becky added, "I try to be positive, but it's not easy." She's aware that I've been going to monasteries but isn't too clear about what that means, except that I'm spending time with people who spend a lot of time in prayer. She writes, "Please ask the monks to pray for me, I need all the help I can get." She responds to a Valentine that my husband and I send her, saying, "Your card made my day. I miss you a lot. I am proud of you and wish my life was busy like yours."

After Becky joined Clubhouse, Dad wrote that while "she finds something every day that becomes a big worry, Clubhouse is good for her. All the clients are people whose mental problems have made them unemployable, and they're trying to get their act together."

The Clubhouse brochure promises a "re-socialization and rehabilitation center for persons with disabling mental illness, offering programs designed to help individuals become more active members of society." The Clubhouse motto reads: "Friendship. A sense of belonging. A place in the community." Becky took those words to heart. Asked for a statement about what Clubhouse meant to her, she had written, "When I feel down I come here and forget my problems. I see new faces and make new friends. We go to good places. I am looking forward to visiting the car wash. I may gain some new knowledge." She enjoyed writing articles for the Clubhouse newsletter, but any disturbance, even a minor spat with another Clubhouse member, would cause her to retreat, and she struggled with regular attendance. She writes, "I mad at me for not going last week."

Becky attends Clubhouse during the week and spends much of each weekend with the family. A part-time volunteer job sorting clothes at a thrift store also gets her out of the house. But incontinence has become an issue, and one day she phones Dad from work, weeping because she wet her pants. She carries enough money to take a taxi in emergencies, but Dad went to get her and take her back to Mrs. R.'s.

As Becky approaches forty, her difficulties are centered less on men than on the women she lives with. By now Becky has been at Mrs. R.'s for eight years, and she frequently quarrels with other residents. "I lost my temper," she writes, "and Mrs. R. yelled at me. I called my shrink and told him I wanted to hurt myself. He put me on a new drug that helped." In her next letter she writes, "I sorry that I wrote that last letter to you when I was depressed, But I have news. One of the staff at Clubhouse said she could see how much I've improved, and I seem happier. It made me cry, and I felt overwhelmed."

About her group home she writes, "I have improved over time, but except for my roommate I don't have friends there. No one to talk to, and Mrs. R. is very busy caring for us." She often has a hard time getting to sleep and is plagued by nightmares and flashbacks. "When that happens I lie awake and try not to make noise. I feel sad," she writes, "but I pray and my angels help me out."

Becky explains to me that she's had limited success in explaining to Mrs. R. why she often shouts at other residents. "I tell Mrs. R.," she writes, "that people get on my nerves, and when I get nervous I get loud."

Becky thinks she's found a solution: "Now," she explains, "when I feel like yelling at people, I write them a note instead." But Mrs. R. tells her that the other residents are annoyed by her letters and find them confusing. Becky doesn't understand and tells me these notes are "my way of dealing with problems." She becomes jealous when another resident gets her own phone, something our family refuses to provide for her. "I turn my radio up to drown out her talking," she writes, adding, "Please don't ask me about my group home."

"I HAVE A HARD TIME LOVING MYSELF"

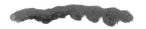

BECKY RECEIVED A LIFELINE when she began to get medical and psychiatric care at Kōkua Kalihi Valley, a community health center that treats people regardless of their ability to pay. Her treatment plan included regular checkups with a physician as well as monthly sessions with a counselor and consultation with a psychiatrist every three months. Her counselor—I'll call her Joyce—is a clinical nurse specialist, much like a nurse practitioner but with an emphasis on mental health. Becky tells me that she decided on meeting her that she could trust her, and the counselor's notes from their first meeting reveal the Becky I knew:

> She reports she is close with family; didn't sleep well last night, nervous about this appt. Feels happy and safe at the group home. But feels confused about her life and doesn't know what she wants. Discussed two incidents of being molested as a child/ preteen and several bad relationships with men. Reported having flashbacks about these incidents at night, says I hate myself when I have the flashbacks. People think I'm friendly but actually I'm shy. She is worried about her brother-in-law David who is being treated for lung cancer.

I'm not sure how honest Becky was with Joyce about her behavior. Our mother had told me and Charlotte that she was sometimes afraid of Becky: as she was growing older, Becky was still strong and given to angry rants. That's probably the reason she didn't go after Becky one day when after visiting the family's Mānoa Valley house, Becky ran off with Mom's purse. Mom phoned Charlotte in a panic, and Charlotte rushed from work downtown. Finding Becky at a bus stop near our house, she jumped the curb, barely missing the bus stop. Grabbing the purse from Becky, she hit her with it and took it back to our mother. Becky later apologized, but Mom and Charlotte remained on alert.

Joyce's written notes indicate that Becky was willing to admit to sometimes hurting others. She was eager to state her goals for improvement. She wanted

to do chores without being told to do them; to decrease the depression resulting from the flashbacks; to have more friends and activities outside the home. Current major problems: I am teased and misunderstood when I talk; I was teased as a child, called a "retard" and I get angry. I have anger problems. I hit other residents. I am too easily irritated. I feel bad when I hurt others. I want to be more independent. I have a hard time loving myself.

"I CAN ONLY CHANGE ME"

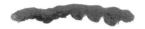

JOYCE NOTED THAT BECKY tended to enter their sessions tense, anxious, angry, and desperate to unload. Then as Joyce listened, Becky would calm down. This description of Becky would be familiar to anyone who knew her well. Our movie dates often began the same way, with tears or a diatribe, and then Becky would gradually relax enough to have a good time.

At the group home, nightmares and flashbacks relating to her sexual molestation often caused Becky to wake up angry in the morning and take out her frustrations on those around her. Becky told her counselor that she couldn't explain to Mrs. R. that one reason she so intensely disliked another resident was because her voice reminded her of the man who had molested her aboard the *Lurline*. "She'd just think it was an excuse," she said. She was reluctant to discuss the molestation with anyone but Joyce.

Everyone in the family knew that Becky sometimes made up stories to feel important or get sympathy, but she demonstrated many of the symptoms associated with being sexually molested as a preteen: anger, antisocial behavior, anxiety, bedwetting, compulsive lying, depression, difficulty establishing intimate relationships, flashbacks, impulsive sexuality, insomnia, low self-image, and nightmares.

A clinical psychologist has told me that flashbacks are a common feature of PTSD, a way of reliving a terrible experience in an attempt to take control of it. But he said they also contribute to a person's low self-esteem; you hate yourself because you couldn't control things in the original experience and allowed bad things to happen to you.

In her notes, Joyce says that while Becky was reluctant to admit to aggressive and inappropriate behavior, she also had good insight into her condition. Joyce's focusing on Becky's strengths seems to have helped my sister better understand what triggered her anger, and how to take responsibility for her actions. In a journal entry about a particular group home resident with whom she'd been feuding, Becky wrote, "When I get angry I can only change me."

"I PASSED THE DRUNK TEST!"

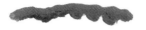

MY SISTER HAD a complex relationship with physicians and often tried to manipulate them. If she was prescribed a medication she didn't like, she'd learn all she could about its side effects and claim to have enough of them that the doctor would take her off the drug. In the many groups Becky attended over the years—anger management, stress management, behavioral therapy—Becky had determined that the adult children of alcoholics got a lot of sympathy. In what I consider a crowning achievement, she convinced a psychiatrist that our mom was a raging alcoholic. The truth was that Mom drank a bit of crème de menthe once or twice a year after a restaurant meal. The psychiatrist made an appointment to see my father, and when the doctor expressed sympathy over his wife's drinking problem, Dad said he'd never laughed so hard in his life. He had difficulty convincing the doctor that he'd been conned.

In her later years, Becky was fortunate in the many physicians who looked after her: a family practice doctor and psychiatrist, a gastroenterologist, a neurologist. Becky enjoyed her annual visits to the neurologist because just as a police officer watches a suspected drunk driver attempt to walk in a straight line, this doctor would observe Becky as she walked around his office. Afterward Becky would cheerfully report, "I passed the drunk test!" She found this an especially good joke because she had stopped drinking alcohol many years before.

Becky was not shy about asking doctors for what she felt she needed. She once wrote a letter to her internist stating, "I need more lab work, a physical exam, and a pap smear." She was probably right. I'm amazed that although Becky was on Medicaid, and her only income came from Social Security disability checks, her doctors treated her as if she were a millionaire. I don't know if that was Hawaii's celebrated Aloha Spirit in action or because the physicians at Kōkua Kalihi Valley took a special interest in her.

Becky would sometimes ask me to come with her when she had two appointments back-to-back: a session with Joyce, her gentle, wise counselor, followed by a more perfunctory visit with the psychiatrist who had a brusque manner of speaking. After one session I asked Becky, "Do you realize they're playing good cop/bad cop with you?" When I explained the principle, Becky seemed surprised. But the next time we saw the psychiatrist she told her, "I know you're the bad cop, and Joyce is the good cop, but I need both of you."

PART FIVE

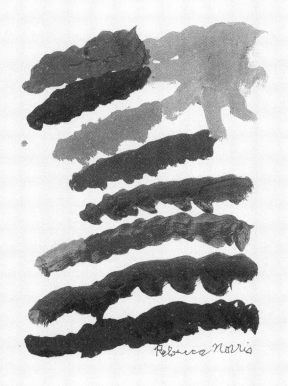

"What Will Happen to Me If You, Dad, and Mom Get Sick?"

"I FEEL HURT BECAUSE YOU WROTE A BOOK AND I DIDN'T"

I TRY NOT TO INDULGE in what-if scenarios, but with my sister it was difficult not to wonder what Becky would have accomplished had she not suffered brain damage during birth. Becky lived with a strong sense of regret that could turn into resentment and jealousy, especially of me. Sometimes she expressed this openly, blurting, "I wish I had found a husband like you did."

When my book *Dakota* was published she sent me this letter:

Dear Kathy,

I feel hurt because you wrote a book and I didn't. Happy for you and I try to read your book and I was bored with it. Mom and dad and everybody talking about it. I feel left out but it will pass. Hope you understand how I feel about your book. I telling you how I feel and I starting to cry while I write this letter.

I suspect many writers wish they had siblings who could express their unease so openly. It can't be easy to have a writer in the family. It can't be easy to have a sister who writes a bestselling book, especially if all of your life you've felt excluded from the party. One great thing about Becky is that she put it all out there—the jealousy, the bafflement over why people were making a big deal about something her annoying sister wrote—and oh, I love her, and it's making me cry to admit all of this.

Becky was in her early forties when *Dakota* was published. One might expect that by that time she'd learned the guile that most of us employ in social relations. But she was like Adam and Eve before the Fall, with no idea that she should hide her more unsavory feelings, unable to pretend that all was well while fierce emotions raged within.

"YOU SHOULD WRITE
A BOOK ABOUT ME"

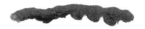

ONCE WHEN BECKY GOT aspiration pneumonia, she had exploratory gastrointestinal surgery, during which a large hiatal hernia was found. I sat with my parents, who were then in their early eighties, in the waiting room during the lengthy operation. When the surgeon came out he said, "The good news is that we didn't find cancer." He added, "But we almost lost her." My mother gasped, and the doctor continued. "She has a strong constitution and she'll be okay. But it will be a long recovery."

We were able to see Becky briefly in the surgical recovery room, but my parents were distressed to see her hooked up to so many medical devices. Becky squeezed our hands but was unable to talk due to the tubes in her throat. The nurse reassured us that the tubes would be taken out when Becky was stronger, and so far her vital signs were good. I promised my parents that I'd visit Becky every day and give them updates.

One day as I was about to enter Becky's room with a small teddy bear I intended to give her, a nurse stopped me and said that it would be better if I didn't go in. He said that Becky had become extremely agitated after my last visit. "Do you know why?" he asked, glaring at me, as if I must be guilty of treating my sister badly. I was surprised and told him that I did a lot for Becky. I guess this is just old sister stuff, I said. He looked doubtful. I added that my parents were counting on me to report on how she was doing, but I could stop at the nurses' station to avoid upsetting Becky. I was hoping I'd be able to see her in a few days.

When Becky suddenly suffered respiratory arrest, she was intubated again and moved back to intensive care. She eventually pulled through and soon was speaking with pride about having to take "swallowing tests" and to drink something no one in the family had heard of, thickened water. And as much as she enjoyed eating, she was less worried than I when her doctor determined that for a time she would need a PEG tube, a gastric feeding tube in a small slit in the abdomen that goes directly into the stomach. This meant that she could not go back to her group home immediately but would stay in a nursing home for a time.

At the home, Becky typically made the best of the situation, attempting to make friends with the staff and other patients, although many were unable to communicate verbally. The aides were pleasant but incompetent and allowed Becky's incision to become infected, a potentially life-threatening condition. Her gastroenterologist, a fierce advocate for his patients, threatened to remove Becky from their care and put her back in the hospital until she was ready to go home.

Becky was strongly motivated to get well and regain some measure of independence. I was encouraged by her steady progress, relieved to see her returning to form, and enjoying all the attention she was receiving. We began to talk about what movies we would see when she was better.

Becky had begun to think that my success as a writer could benefit her. One day she said, "You should write a book about me, so I can be famous like you." But I could not forget that when my sister was in the ICU she had not been able to stand the sight of me. I'll always wonder if that was because in my life she could see an image of what hers could have been.

THE WRITER IN THE FAMILY

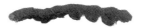

I WOULDN'T BE SURPRISED if Becky was meant to be a writer, most likely a novelist, as she possessed a marked gift for invention. She had learned early on that if you tell people what they want to hear, they will like you. And as getting people on her side was Becky's major motivator, she became a fabulist, a habitual liar.

Becky had difficulty grasping that her falsehoods could hurt people. Her habit of stretching the truth was especially hard on Charlotte when she was young. Children tend to accept the world as it's presented and can have difficulty discerning falsehood.

When I asked my nieces how old they were when they realized that much of what Becky said was a fabrication, one recalled that if her mother overheard what Becky was telling her, she'd take her aside and say, "That's not true; it's just how Becky talks." Another replied that she trusted her Aunt Becky but was about seven years old when she realized that other members of the family did not, and often treated Becky more like a child than an adult.

Joyce had told me that from the time my sister began seeing her, Becky claimed to have a steady boyfriend. She would talk about how handsome he was and all the places he'd taken her in his nice car. When she said, "He's not allowed to enter my group home, so no one there knows him; my parents don't know him either," Joyce realized the man was a fantasy. She didn't challenge Becky, as apparently conjuring this man was one way Becky had found to assuage her loneliness.

While Becky could make rational decisions, she never outgrew an inability to distinguish between fantasy and reality. This, along with her need to send stream-of-consciousness letters to everyone she knew, is one reason I've long felt that she was meant to be the writer in the family.

HO'OMALIMALI

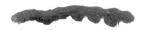

HO'OMALIMALI IS A HAWAIIAN word for flattery, often used when people sense that there's insincerity and an ulterior motive behind the pleasing words a person is saying.

Charlotte tells me that Becky would often ask her for advice about boyfriends, money, clothing, and hair styles. And while Becky thanked her profusely—"Oh you understand me, you give me the best advice"—she would then ignore what Charlotte had said. In calling Becky's effusive gratitude *ho'omalimali*, she wasn't implying that Becky had a malicious intent; she knew it was her way of trying to make Charlotte feel that she valued her opinions.

Becky's habit of taking you aside and whispering something in a conspiratorial manner was also *ho'omalimali*. She was trying to make you feel special by letting you in on a secret; it made her feel important, someone with vital information to impart. But Becky's *ho'omalimali* combined with her disregard for the truth could have unfortunate consequences.

When Charlotte's young children were reeling from the news that she was divorcing their father, I overhead Becky tell them, "I think they're getting back together." It was the worst thing she could have said and came at the worst possible time. I was angry at Becky and told her so. When I told Charlotte, she became angry as well; she would now have to raise the painful subject of the impending divorce with her confused children yet again and try to undo the damage Becky had done. We understood that Becky was unaware of the harm she was doing. She knew the children wanted their parents to stay together and thought it was important for them to believe that this was possible.

This was one of many occasions when I wanted to scream at Becky but didn't. I did try to convey to her that it was unfair to the children to get their hopes up, because their parents' marriage was over. But Becky didn't want to believe that. Marriage was sacred to her, and as with her imaginary boyfriend, what Becky dreamed of and wished for was better than the reality.

"I WAS PRAYING FOR THAT"

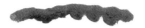

THE FAMILY, EVEN THE CHILDREN, learned to take Becky's exaggerations and falsehoods in stride. We let her get away with her more harmless fancies, such as her tendency to say that her prayers came true. Whenever something good happened—a niece was accepted by the college of her choice, I got a poem published—Becky would respond by saying, "I was praying for that." I'm convinced that Becky believed in the efficacy of prayer, even when hers weren't answered in the way she wanted, something she occasionally complained about. But she also enjoyed the attention she received by claiming that something good had come about through her prayers.

Becky adored Father Michael, the young associate priest at my Episcopal church, in no small part because when I was out of town he sometimes enlisted the aid of a woman parishioner to take Becky to a movie. When he visited her at home, he'd bring her a Diet Coke. These acts meant the world to Becky.

Once when she was in a hospital recovering from pneumonia, Father Michael visited and Becky told him she was lonely; it had been years since she'd been on a date. He replied that he felt much the same way. He was new in town and was hoping to find someone special who would share his life.

Becky said, "Yes; I've been praying that you'll find a lover." Michael was startled but recovered enough to reply, "Thank you, Becky, for thinking of me."

Becky sent Father Michael a thank-you card after each movie excursion and hospital visit. It was typical of her to make cards out of construction paper and illustrate them with drawings of flowers, hearts, and stars. She'd add notes in crayon; large, unwieldy letters expressing raw emotion in a flow of prose that said more about her than the person being addressed. Mom was a frequent recipient.

One Valentine as Becky wrote it reads: "Mom, Happy Valentine Day—I'vd a confession to make with you, I took $10.00 out of your purse but I pay you back Here is $10.00 I love you. I may be moving to nursing home I happy to talk about it."

A card she made for our mother for her seventieth birthday reads:

Happy to a woman is younger and wise own way Happy Brith Day. You're getting wisdom—wise your age. Thank you for bring me in this world. I'd accept it but it took long time—I deal with it You understand me better then my siblings. You're only 35 old today or as young as you want be.

Love, Special Daughter

Becky

"I DON'T WANT MOM OR DAD TO DIE"

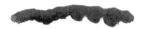

BECKY'S ABILITY TO GET to the heart of things could be startling. One year when David and I had come for the holidays, Becky and I left the house and went for a walk on Christmas Eve in Mānoa Valley. She was extremely anxious and when I asked her what was wrong, she blurted, "I don't want Mom and Dad to die. I worry about what will happen to me."

This was the first time Becky had expressed this concern to me. I replied, "It scares me too," adding, "but I think it frightens everyone to think about their parents dying." Becky seemed surprised; she tended to think she suffered such fears alone.

Our parents had always been strong advocates for Becky, and now she harbored the reasonable suspicion that her sisters, brother, and sister-in-law might not be up to the task of looking out for her in the same dogged way. I tried to convince her that even after our mother and father were gone, we would still take care of her.

We were two middle-aged women whose parents had entered their eighties. Two women, one considered mentally slow and one fast by comparison, acknowledging the fact that one day in the not too distant future we would be orphans.

In Mānoa Valley it rains somewhere nearly every day. Winter can bring torrential downpours. But on that day the rain was so light it barely moistened our skin, making it shine like gold in the sunlight. I told Becky that anyone looking in our direction would see a rainbow, and that cheered her up.

"I'M ACTING LIKE A CHILD, AND I DON'T KNOW WHY"

THE DEFINITION OF *NORMAL* in *The American Heritage Dictionary*, 3rd Edition, reads in part: "relating to or characterized by average intelligence and development . . . free from emotional disorder."

1. "CHARACTERIZED BY AVERAGE INTELLIGENCE AND DEVELOPMENT"

When it came to intelligence, Becky was hard to place. Just as often as she would confound you with a lack of understanding she could demonstrate great acuity and wisdom.

Becky's IQ was ranked in the low 90s. But that number was not particularly useful with regard to Becky. She had an exceptional memory. A physician who saw her regularly told me that Becky would pick up where their previous conversation left off, as if several months hadn't elapsed. And she'd recall every detail of that earlier conversation, which meant that if you made a promise to Becky, you had better be prepared to keep it.

Becky also took keen interest in her health and became so knowledgeable about her medications that her longtime counselor at Kōkua Kalihi Valley had her give talks to other patients at medication management sessions.

My sister knew what happened to her if she didn't take her medications. One Christmas Eve she walked into an emergency room and said she was having a crisis, as she'd been deceiving her family and group home operator and hadn't taken her psych meds for over a week. When a nurse phoned me, I went immediately to the hospital. When Becky saw me she wept and said, "I've been acting like a child, and I don't know why." I told the physician that I saw my sister's aberrant behavior as a somewhat normal-if-panicked response to the fact that it's Christmas, always a stressful time for her; and it was especially difficult this year, as our father was dying. He'd had aplastic anemia for years, but its symptoms were becoming more severe. He had told the family that he knew this would be his last Christmas.

The doctor's notes read: "Reports some falls, is slightly disoriented but responsive to counseling. Discussed that if she's admitted to the hospital she may not be accepted back into care home due to non-compliance and decompensating. Also reports feeling guilty over the effects of her behavior on her father's health."

I was able to take my sister back to Mrs. R.'s later that day, but Becky's intuition that something was seriously wrong proved correct. While her caregiver had regarded her bedwetting and coughing with vomiting as regressive misbehavior, Becky was in much more serious condition than anyone, even that emergency room physician, had realized. Not long after she returned home, her caregiver called an ambulance, and Becky was admitted to the hospital, found to have polyuria (excessive urination resulting in excessive sodium in her blood) as well as renal failure. The emergency room notes read in part:

> During the episodes of coughing/vomiting patient may not have been absorbing psych meds. Delirious and confused. Admitted with aspiration pneumonia and reflux. Primary diagnosis: Aspiration pneumonia, multilobar, probably secondary to severe gastric reflux and Barrett's esophagus. Secondary diagnosis: bronchial washing, positivity for methicillin-resistant staphylococcus aureus; severe

gastro reflux disease; hiatal hernia; Barrett's esophagus; dysphasia; anemia; nephrogenic diabetes insipidus; post-Nissen fundoplication; gastric tube placement; skin candidiasis; post-mechanical intubation; bi-polar disorder; mental retardation; tremors.

Becky is described as "an unfortunate 49 year old woman with multiple medical problems. recurrent aspiration due to severe reflux and esophagitis. Cleared in ER as psychologically stable." Becky may have been "unfortunate" in many ways, but she was so much more. What in the world could "normal" mean in this context?

2. "FREE FROM EMOTIONAL DISORDER"

Anyone who is truly "free from emotional disorder" hasn't been paying attention. Artists and writers often learn to live with the ups and downs on what used to be termed the manic-depressive scale and can learn to live with them. For psychiatrists these terms have specific definitions, but looking at the words they employ in assessing a patient's thought processes—tangential, circumstantial, disorganized, loose, flight of ideas—I'd say that every one of them is useful, if not necessary, in writing a poem.

And so is what a South Dakota friend aptly terms "jackrabbit speech." If you can picture a large hare running in a zigzag pattern, you can appreciate the manner of speech both Becky and I employed. It may seem vague and digressive, but it's a useful method of thought and may be seen as a normal part of the writing process.

When Becky was a child, while she wore her feelings on her sleeve, her emotional responses were fairly normal. We had the usual sibling rivalries and arguments, which meant that Becky had to learn how to fight fair and square and then make up. And we all had to learn when to make allowances for her disability and when to call her out for bad behavior. To outsiders the this may have seemed odd; to us it was normal.

MISFITS

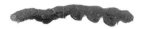

B ECKY HAD BEEN in so many mental health programs at a variety of facilities in Honolulu that she got to know many of the town misfits, the unfortunates you pass by on the streets but often don't acknowledge as people with names or histories. She made me remember that these are the people Jesus encountered and loved, even though their illnesses had made them social outcasts. The Gospels invite us to see Christ in all of them, but we often settle for making a monthly contribution to a homeless shelter.

When we saw a man walking gingerly through town, barefoot and bare-chested, holding shopping bags in each arm as if they were keeping him balanced, Becky told me she had been in a group therapy program with him. Becky knew the stories behind some of the women who walked downtown or at a shopping mall, ranting and screaming, their hair matted, their clothes reeking of urine. She'd whisper to me that one had walked out of a group home and never returned; she knew that another had a series of abusive boyfriends.

One of Becky's roommates at Mrs. R.'s, who told me she'd been diagnosed as severely bipolar, was an educated woman from a wealthy and socially prominent family in Chicago. She had retained her good manners and the social graces: whenever I treated her and Becky to lunch and a movie she would send me a thank-you note in the mail. I enjoyed her company and was grateful that she understood Becky so well. But I had to wonder what had gone so terribly wrong in her life that she was living in a group home in one of Honolulu's poorest neighborhoods.

If Becky had not had our family for support, and if our parents had not been so diligent about seeking help for her, Becky could well have ended up on the street, shouting at strangers, demanding to be heard, but having no one who would listen. Becky knew this; being abandoned and left to fend for herself was her greatest fear.

"I GUESS THIS IS WHAT IT MEANS TO BE BIPOLAR"

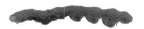

BECKY WAS STUNNED when I told her that my husband, a man she loved, had once described her as one of the angriest people he had ever known. She became uncharacteristically speechless, as this belied the person Becky wanted to present to the world. That Becky was a good person, someone who was always positive and helpful. Becky often repeated this mantra, but those who knew her well could discern the desperation behind it.

When Becky's good cheer failed her, she couldn't control her fall into the abyss. If she greeted me effusively at a medical clinic or movie theater, saying in a tone of exaggerated sweetness, "You're my best sister; you're my angel sister," it was a sure sign that in a few hours she'd become furious with me over some inconsequential thing and shout, "You're my worst sister!"

Becky's anger ran deep. She knew what had happened to her when she was born, and lived every day with the knowledge that she had been irredeemably damaged by a physician's error. Dad once remarked that if Becky's brain injury had been more severe, it might have been appropriate to put her in a care facility. But, he added, if she'd had a little less damage, she could have run for Congress. Becky got it; she laughed at the joke.

One day Becky arrived at the senior living facility where Mom and Dad moved after climbing stairs at the Mānoa Valley house had become too much for them. She was coughing, her voice was raspy, her eyes were red. Our mother had recently been released from the hospital after a bout with pneumonia, and while I was appalled that Becky would have come to Mom's place in this condition, I wasn't surprised. I had promised to take Becky to the movies, and nothing could keep her from that.

I got my sister out of the apartment as quickly as possible and didn't let her near our mother. I finessed that situation, but on another occasion I had to take drastic action. I'd taken Becky to a movie, and as we approached Mom's apartment, Becky's good mood was evaporating fast. She was working herself into a fury for reasons that I doubt even she fully understood.

Mom was then nearly ninety years of age, and I took advantage of my edge in mobility to race to her apartment, enter, and lock the door behind me. When Becky arrived she pounded on the door and shouted, demanding that I let her in. I told her I couldn't until she calmed down; that it wasn't fair to Mom. More pounding and shouting. Then silence, and finally a plaintive, "I'm sorry, please let me in. I'll behave." I opened the door and Becky entered.

Mom was a paragon of unconditional love, and Becky was in full retreat. They sat on the couch and hugged each other and soon were bickering amicably about what television program to watch. Mom told Becky she could choose, and Becky began to smile through her tears. She said, "I guess this is what it means to be bipolar."

"I'LL BE FINE. I HAVE A POSITIVE ATTITUDE"

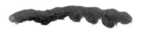

MY SISTER COULD DRIVE YOU to distraction with incessant talk about the importance of being positive. She had picked up the term in group therapy and it stuck. Whatever she had to endure, she would claim that being positive was helping her get through it. And to a large degree this worked for her.

Becky performed a breast self-exam every month, and when she found a lump on one breast, she was aware of the danger it posed and asked to see her doctor immediately. When a biopsy revealed that it was a cancerous tumor, Becky's doctor told me that my sister had fallen through the cracks so often in her life, she was determined that it not happen again. She got Becky the best possible care, referring her to the surgeon who had treated Hawaii's governor, Linda Lingle, for breast cancer.

On the day Becky began treatment following her breast cancer surgery, I felt uneasy walking from my condo to meet Becky at the treatment center. It was the last place I wanted to be, as it was exactly a week after my husband had died in the intensive care unit of another Honolulu hospital. But Becky had said she needed me there because "you know all about this hospital stuff."

It was Halloween, and when we entered the clinic, we found that the nurses were in costume. One wore a colorful clown outfit, one had her face painted like a cat, another wore a witch's hat and a broom pin next to her name tag. The nurse who presented our orientation told Becky, "We did this all just for you," which I think Becky half-believed.

This nurse told us what Becky could expect. Nausea was likely, but the first drug Becky would take that day would help with that. Eventually Becky would experience hair loss, anemia, and fatigue, but the woman reassured us that as these symptoms surfaced, they could provide medication to ease them.

She then showed us a small refrigerator that contained sandwiches, fresh fruit, and sodas, and told Becky that she could request food and drink at any time. Becky's eyes grew wide; she began to see this place as a refuge from her group home. She became even happier when we went to the treatment station, where a large, comfortable recliner faced a picture window with a view of trees and the lawn of the Shriner's Children's Hospital across the street. There was also a small television set. "This is your personal TV," the nurse said, "and you can watch anything you like." Becky exclaimed, "Oh, goodie!" In her group home there were often arguments over the television, with one set available for four women. Once Becky had gotten into trouble with Mrs. R. and her social worker for hitting another resident with a remote control. Mrs. R. had resolved the conflict by giving each woman control of the remote one day a week.

When the nurse asked Becky how she was feeling about receiving chemotherapy she said, firmly: "I'll be fine. I have a positive attitude." And while I often sensed a forced bravado in my sister, a paper-thin mask over a chasm of despair, I have to respect her ability to face frightening circumstances with a good spirit.

Over the next few months, Becky and I settled into a routine. I'd walk to the hospital to meet her, and in the treatment room I'd find her favorite TV channel so she could watch programs from her childhood:

Gunsmoke or *Leave It to Beaver*. She'd send me to the refrigerator for sandwiches and soft drinks. Sometimes she would whisper to me about other patients who seemed depressed. After her treatment was over we often went to a movie.

Anemia eventually set in, and Becky complained about feeling tired all the time. "You need to tell the nurses," I said, reminding her that on our first visit we'd been told that she'd eventually become fatigued and could ask for medication to help with that. When Becky began to lose her hair, she charged me with finding turbans, instructing me to find ones in bright colors, with sequins if possible. She was offered a free wig from a charity and happily settled on a cute pageboy in an ash-blond shade. When we were at a restaurant or a movie theater, she would point to me, grin broadly, and announce to a waiter or ticket taker, "I'm her only blond sister!"

"I THINK YOU'RE RIGHT"

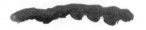

AFTER HER TREATMENT for breast cancer ended, Becky said she wanted me to take her to Disneyland. We had gone there as a family in 1965 when Becky was thirteen. She had loved the Alice in Wonderland ride and didn't mind getting dizzy as we rode in spinning teacups. The highlight for her was the boat ride underneath the castle she'd seen on the weekly Disney television show.

Becky often said she was jealous of all the travel I did; she felt left out, especially when I was able to add a family visit to a business trip and see one of our nieces on the mainland. When I sent her postcards from the cities I visited on book tours, she complained that she was stuck in a group home. I thought she deserved something special after her cancer treatments but felt that it wouldn't be wise for us to attempt a trip to Disneyland.

Becky sometimes made it difficult to do nice things for her. After her chemo ended and her hair grew back, I asked her if she'd like my hairdresser to style it. She readily agreed, so I set up an appointment and arranged for a cab driver to pick Becky up at her care home. I was to meet her at the salon and take her to lunch afterward, so she could show off her new hairdo. I was surprised when the driver called to say that when he arrived at Becky's place she sent him away, saying she didn't feel like going out. I paid him for his trouble and called the hairdresser to apologize for the last-minute cancelation.

I was angry but also relieved, as this incident made it clear that traveling with Becky was out of the question. I could envision her having a tantrum and refusing to board a plane or leave a hotel room. It was too great a risk. Becky, bless her, was receptive when I voiced my concerns. I realized that as she matured, she was becoming more self-aware. I said that if we were able to travel with other family members it might work, but I didn't think she was stable enough to make a trip like that with me. Becky sighed and said, "I think you're right."

PART SIX

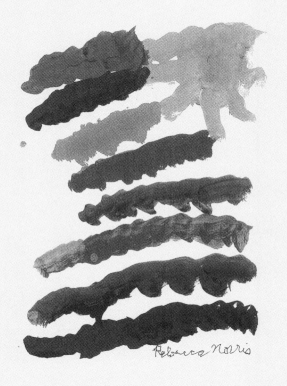

Rebecca Norris

"It's Important to Be the Right Kind of Person"

"A HUGGING CHURCH"

"Needy" is a label I suspect we often use to justify turning away from people who remind us of what it means to be vulnerable. Throughout her life, Becky had been dismissed as needy by people she longed to befriend. She'd pursue them too aggressively and say inappropriate things that caused them to spurn her. Becky was used to being shunned, and this is one reason she enjoyed attending my Episcopal church, where she found acceptance. When she was in her fifties it became an important part of her life.

For years the church sponsored a Thanksgiving meal, providing the turkey, mashed potatoes, and stuffing while parish members contributed side dishes and desserts. We put up signs in nearby apartment buildings, attracting residents of a YWCA halfway house for women recently released from prison, as well as many older neighbors whose children lived far away.

One year this dinner was canceled on short notice. I wanted to share the day with my sister but knew that on a holiday it could be difficult to arrange for rides to and from Becky's group home. I also thought Becky might be reluctant to go to a crowded restaurant. Another church member helped us solve our dilemma.

He was an intelligent man who was decidedly needy, tending to overshare in discussing his many "issues"—mental and physical ailments, dysfunctional family relationships, difficulties in proving that he qualified for an emotional support dog. Like my sister he lived on disability income. Like my sister he used the Handi-Van. He offered to make the van reservations for both of them on Thanksgiving Day. I suggested a popular, reasonably priced restaurant and reserved our places for its holiday buffet.

As usual, Becky didn't feel able to navigate the buffet line. "You know what I like," she said, "you go for me." Emphatically she added, "No rice!" She was served rice every day at home and was looking forward to potatoes. She laughed when I told her I'd get her mashed potatoes, scalloped potatoes, sweet potatoes, Okinawan potatoes, any kind of potatoes I could find.

This day was more joyful than I had expected. I encountered a high school classmate who showed me photographs of her grandchildren. Becky and our friend had a long conversation about church, growing up in Hawaii, and their experience of psychiatrists, psychologists, and psychotropic medications. When he went to get second helpings, Becky whispered in astonishment, "Kathy, he takes more meds than I do!"

I said, "Well, Becky, you've talked with him long enough to realize that he needs them." She nodded and said, "He's crazier than I am." I replied, "You may be right, but I don't know what we would have done today without him." Becky nodded.

When I think of Becky's neediness, I think of all the love she had to offer, as witnessed by her ability to care for severely disabled children when she was young and the gift for friendship that emerged in her maturity. It grieves me that she never found work as a nurse's aide or met a partner with whom she could share her love. It made me glad to see how readily she took to being loved by the people of my parish. She dubbed it "a hugging church."

"I KNOW NOW PEOPLE LIVE AND DIE"

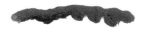

IN JUNE OF 2002, after Dad suffered what one physician characterized as a "major metabolic disturbance" following a blood transfusion for his worsening aplastic anemia, his kidneys began to fail. Rather than put him through more invasive procedures, the family got him out of the hospital and into home hospice at the senior living facility.

We told Becky Dad was dying and made sure she could spend time with him. In a journal entry from that week Becky wrote: "I know now people live and die. Before I thought live forever. Yesterday I told dad sorry all the trouble I cause you."

I can still see Becky standing by Dad's bed and taking his hand. "Dad," she said, "I'm sorry for all the times I was bad and made you worry. I tried to do better, but couldn't always do it. I'm sorry. I love you, please forgive me." When Becky turned to us, we told her that we were sure he had heard what she said, even if he couldn't respond. She nodded and we shared a group hug, all of us in tears.

The next morning my brother and I went to tell Becky that Dad had died a few hours after she saw him. Becky wrote in her journal that day: "My dad went, he really died. Went peaceful without any pain, go to Heaven. You'll be missed cause I'll miss father daughter talks, since I special." Plaintively, she adds, "It is still hard to love me; my best friend was dad. There are times I cry about this. How to deal with it?"

Becky reports to her counselor Joyce, "I talked to my dad on Friday and that night he died." Over the next few months Becky experienced episodes of weeping, feeling dizzy, and acting out at home, throwing one resident's plate of food to the floor, pushing another against the kitchen sink. Joyce asks Becky to enroll in an anger management class and keep an anger journal in which she will keep track of the times when she feels like she's losing control. Within a few months Joyce reports that Becky seems better able to live with her grief. I was taking her to movies at least once a week, and that helped us both. Over lunch we'd share memories of our father.

When Joyce suggested that Becky engage in volunteer work, Becky said she wanted to work again with disabled children. Her application to work at a Ronald McDonald House was rejected, and she wrote in her journal that this made her cry. But she also set goals for herself: "to make more friends, to be nicer to my caregiver and other residents, to practice coping skills, and try not to argue but ask for time out when I'm angry."

Our father's death caused Becky to dwell on the circumstances of her birth, and she wrote to me that she's never felt that she belonged in this world. "Been crying about the doctor who let me down when I was little," she writes, "cause I didn't have enough oxygen to my head. Like I didn't want to come out at all, like it wasn't my time yet."

"I NEED TO SPREAD MY WINGS"

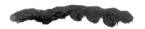

BECKY WAS STILL LIVING at Mrs. R.'s when Dad's death triggered a round of angry behavior, with Becky acting aggressively toward other residents at her group home. A year later, when Becky received her diagnosis of breast cancer and had surgery followed by radiation and chemotherapy, it added considerably to Becky's stress and acting out.

Becky's breast cancer had not spread to her lymph nodes, and while there were episodes of yelling at Mrs. R.'s during her six months of treatment, she came through in good shape, both physically and mentally. But after Becky recovered, Mrs. R. told Becky's social worker and Joyce that she could no longer handle Becky's moodiness. Becky had been regressing, and as she'd been in the care home much longer than any of the other residents, she'd become increasingly territorial. She was especially hard on newcomers.

Becky herself was eager for a move. She's been telling the family and her counselor that she's bored at home and wants to enroll in a day program. She tells Joyce, "I need to spread my wings; I need a change." John and Marilyn, who were planning to move to the mainland within a year, worked with a social worker on finding a new placement for Becky and settled on one run by a middle-aged couple with years of experience in running a group home.

They proved to be diligent in their record keeping and getting Becky to her medical appointments, but she wasn't happy in their home. The caregivers kept the refrigerator in the downstairs area locked and became upset with Becky when she found a way to steal sodas. Becky complained to us that she and the other residents were placed in a separate room whenever the family had a party or birthday celebration, and my family could not convince the caregivers to let us know in advance so that Becky could spend that time with us.

We began to notice that whenever we had taken Becky on a pleasant outing, the closer we got to this group home, the more agitated and angry she became. By the time we got to the driveway, she'd rapidly exit the car, tell us to go to hell, and slam the door.

We understood that Becky had good reason to be frustrated. She couldn't live on her own and resented needing help with the basics of daily life. She was usually much more intelligent than her roommates, and sometimes the caregivers themselves. They were not mean people—my family would have been attuned to any abuse—but the atmosphere they provided could be dispiriting.

"SHE APPEARS OLDER THAN HER STATED AGE"

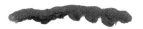

IT WAS DIFFICULT TO WATCH Becky's physical decline in her later years, as she went from walking on her own to relying on a cane, then using a walker, and finally needing a wheelchair. She'd been an active child, an enthusiastic if flailing swimmer. The family has films of Becky as a girl falling sideways into pools, in awkward attempts at diving. She never mastered any stroke beyond the dog paddle. But no matter; she had loved being in the water.

I tried to convince Becky that she and I could exercise together in the heated pool at our mother's senior facility. Becky seemed dubious. I told her that simply walking in the warm water could help her a great deal. She wouldn't have to swim, just walk. Mom had a swimsuit that she thought would fit Becky, but when she put it on and saw herself in the mirror, she frowned and began taking it off, too self-conscious to wear it in public.

As a young adult Becky was an inveterate walker. When she first moved into Mrs. R.'s in the Kalihi neighborhood of Honolulu, she easily navigated a long, steep hill from the bus stop when she returned home after visiting the family. But when Becky was in her fifties, hernia surgery and repeated hospitalizations for a variety of infections took a toll. Hospital notes from that time tell a sad story. Just three months after her hernia surgery, she is readmitted to the hospital with a kidney infection. Her past use of lithium had evidently caused her to develop nephrogenic diabetes insipidus, a rare kidney disease that seems like the Catch-22 of conditions, as it causes both excessive urination and excessive thirst. I believe this is the reason that over the years Becky's caregivers often complained about her stealing sodas. She'd been thirsty and most likely wasn't being provided with adequate hydration because of her incontinence.

During one hospital stay, Becky had such severe tremors she could not feed herself. A physician noted that Becky was "alert and had incomprehensible dysarthric speech; could occasionally follow a simple command. Could not sit up, even with maximal assistance. Could not give medical history; got it from her sister who was there." Becky remained in the hospital for several weeks, and after she was released, John and I hired a physical therapist to work with Becky several times a week at our mom's apartment. Even though Becky reported having felt paranoid while she was in the hospital, after her release her counselor at Kōkua Kalihi Valley found her lucid and alert with no sign of disordered thought.

A few months after completing her cancer treatments, Becky returned to the Queen's Hospital emergency room on her own, reporting that she was unable to control her weeping and bad moods. The physician's notes read: "Highly agitated, crying spells, at high risk for depression." He sent her home with a referral to their outpatient mental health program.

Becky continued to see Joyce once a month but soon was complaining about feeling weak. She'd fallen several times and said that activity often made her short of breath. As usual, Becky was correct about her condition. She was diagnosed with pneumonia, the first of several cases over the next two years. The admitting doctor's notes on one of those hospitalizations reads like a horror story:

Acute pneumonia with sepsis; reconditioning; UTI, pancyto-penia; acute renal failure, resolved; hypocalcemia, resolved;

bi-polar, essential tremor, GTI with Barretts; IgE; immuno-deficiency; Colonization with MRSA. Appears to get pancy-topenia with any infection, but improves with antibiotics; some mood swings and hallucinations; iron deficiency anemia, hyperlipidemia—started on Lipitor, improved.

On this occasion Becky remained hospitalized for two months and was then released to the facility's nursing home for rehabilitation. She remained there for another two months and enjoyed the social life there so much she wanted to remain. But after Becky was assessed by a hospital physician, a social worker told me that Becky did not yet qualify for a higher level of care. This meant finding a new group home, one that could accommodate Becky's need for a walker. She was fifty-six years old, but the hospital notes indicate that "she appears older than her stated age."

"NO ONE LOVES YOU; YOU SHOULD JUST DIE"

BECKY HEARD VOICES and was often compelled to respond to them. When my brother and Marilyn would drive Becky home from a movie or a family dinner, she'd sit in the back seat and carry on a conversation with nonexistent people. But she knew not to do this when her two young nieces were in the car.

One day Becky's caregiver called me to say that Becky had become so agitated she had called an ambulance. When I met Becky in the Queen's emergency room, I found her extremely confused and belligerent. The hospital didn't want to admit her, but I refused to take her home. "You know she'll just be back in a few hours," I said to a harried nurse, feeling a little belligerent myself. The nurse said she'd see what she could do and returned, offering us a session with a hospital social worker. I asked Becky, "Does this sound good to you?" She nodded.

I forget exactly what that social worker said, but Becky soon relaxed and began talking sensibly again. She had simply needed another person to hear her out. When she told the man she was hearing voices more often than usual he asked, "What do they say to you?" Becky replied that it was always terrible things: "No one loves you, you should just die, no one cares what happens to you." "Do they ask you to hurt yourself?" he asked, and she said, "Sometimes," adding, "but I know they're not real." At this I entered the conversation and said,

"Becky, if you know they're not real, you've won half the battle." The social worker nodded in agreement. I added, "If you know they aren't real, you can tell them to go to hell, where they belong. I'm not going to worry about this anymore."

Becky began to laugh. I said, "If you're feeling OK, why don't we go to a movie before I take you home?" I found an inane comedy with a good dose of slapstick. Becky ate her popcorn, drank her soda, and all was well.

VOWS

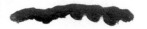

THE VOWS ONE TAKES when becoming a Benedictine oblate are like marriage vows in that you make them in faith without having any idea of what they will demand of you. I became an oblate at forty, when during a Mass, I stood at an altar surrounded by monks who had become my friends and mentors, and promised that according to my situation in life, I would maintain stability of heart, fidelity to the spirit of the monastic way of life, and obedience to the will of God.

"Oh, is that all?" asked a mocking voice within, before I tamped it down. Over subsequent years I have come to know much more about what that "all" entails and am grateful that the vows have acted as spiritual counselors, a firm standard by which to understand and respond to what is happening in my life.

The vows came to the fore when I unexpectedly became a caregiver for my husband. I feared that I wouldn't be much good at it, but in tending to David as he was beset by a number of serious medical issues, my stability became essential. He needed to know he could rely on me, and the vows allowed me to draw on strengths I didn't know I had.

Christianity is a communal faith. You may pray alone but you're a member of the body of Christ. Benedictine life is centered on community, and while my life is much different from that of a person living in a monastery, I take my vow of obedience to God to mean that whatever suffering comes my way, I am simply sharing in the common human lot. Spend some time in the waiting room of an oncology clinic and you'll see what I mean.

Psalm 16 contains one of the most difficult demands in all of Scripture. Verse 6 reads: "The lot marked out for me is my delight, welcome indeed the heritage that falls to me!" If I can pray that from the heart, I'm fulfilling my vow of obedience.

All of this is to say that while the deaths of my father and my husband coming within a year of each other was difficult, my oblate vows helped me to cope. And as my mother became more frail and my sister Becky's medical condition worsened, I had the vows to help me give them the attention and care they required. When the couple operating Becky's group home decided that they could no longer cope with her substantial round of medical appointments, her constant complaining, and unpredictable behavior, my brother and Marilyn were living on the mainland, and it fell to me to find another place for her. At the same time Mom's needs for care were increasing. Although she received assistance from aides with daily medications, showering, and dressing, she depended on me for many things, from helping her change her diapers to getting her to doctor appointments. All of this meant that I was often too exhausted, both physically and mentally, to do much writing. The feeling that I used to be a writer often nagged at me, and I wondered if that vocation was gone for good.

A Benedictine friend once said, "The whole point of monastic life is getting over yourself." Caregiving while remaining faithful to the spirit of monastic life will constantly remind you that whatever emotional burden you're carrying can be dealt with later. Your job is doing whatever needs to be done for your loved one, here and now.

"A SWAN, AND NOT THE UGLY DUCKLING"

BY 2007 BECKY HAD SURVIVED about with cancer and grieving over the deaths of both our father and my husband. She received a great blessing when an emergency room physician referred to an excellent outpatient mental health program at Queen's Hospital. Becky told me that the staff made her "feel like a swan, and not the ugly duckling."

This program did a remarkable job of helping my sister become an adult. Its staff recognized something about Becky that I had learned years before. She was capable of maturing, but it took a long time. I told the staff that Becky's worst behavior had diminished as she got older, but she still clung to the narcissism that I felt she'd developed as a defense mechanism.

I added that this narcissism had surfaced recently in a conversation with my sister. I'd been trying to give Becky news about a recent event in my life—I forget now what it was, but it was important me at the time—when she interrupted: "No," she said; "I go first. My story is more important than yours!"

I said that I had resisted the temptation to laugh but had marveled at Becky's gift for saying out loud what most people have the sense to keep to themselves. She laid out her self-centeredness so openly and innocently it was hard to be upset with her. Yet Becky was no innocent. She was capable of acting out of anger, spite, or jealousy, but like a child she exhibited these emotions so transparently that it was easy for those who loved her to cope.

PHONE HUGS

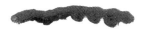

A SOCIAL WORKER ON THE QUEEN'S STAFF told me that when she asked Becky about behavior she wanted to change, she brought up phone conversations with family members. We all knew that Becky enjoyed talking on the phone, but we'd learned to expect that her anger would escalate during a call. Many calls ended with her ranting, cursing, and slamming down the receiver. But Becky had also given the family the "phone hug." During a call, if she felt you were in need of comfort, she'd make an "mmmmm" sound over the phone, as if she were with you, her arms around you. Becky's invention caught on, and for years most family phone conversations ended with phone hugs.

The staff helped Becky compose a written contract, a pledge that reads in part, "Becky has agreed to respond in the following manner when she doesn't want to converse on the phone: 'I don't feel like talking right now. I will call you later to let you know how I am.' Becky has agreed to respond this way on the phone 3 out of 5 times, and try to end calls with a phone hug."

The woman asked the family to monitor Becky's behavior on the phone and to be sure to praise her when she complied with the agreement. She found Becky's honesty remarkable. "Nearly everyone," she said, "when we ask them how often they'll be able to keep the contract, they say, 100 percent of the time. When we asked Becky that, she thought for a moment, and replied, 'Maybe 75-80 percent.'" I'd say her success rate was closer to 99 percent. After Becky signed that contract, she hung up on me only once. And the next time I saw her, she apologized.

Becky had been a sweet little girl. But her experience of others rejecting or ridiculing her for being "slow" had taught her that being nice didn't get her very far. She became difficult, demanding, stubborn. You ignored my sister at your peril. She was on the defensive for so much of her life that she was well into her fifties before she could make a sincere apology. To settle our childhood squabbles, Mom and Dad sometimes forced Becky to say "I'm sorry," but I detected a hard glint in her eye, a refusal to acknowledge that she'd done anything wrong. So this was progress.

Staff members frequently called to discuss Becky with me, and I told them she often talked about how happy she was there. She was especially proud that she'd learned to cook scrambled eggs for the group. But as the staff was teaching Becky new skills, they were also assessing her and asked me to fill them in on Becky's history. I said that in my experience the clearest indication of my sister's brain damage was her innumeracy. Being unable to comprehend the value of money had caused trouble in the past, as Becky was an easy target for anyone wanting to take advantage of her. They might ask for a dollar, or twenty dollars, and Becky wouldn't know the difference.

I told them that I had recently met Becky at a movie theater, and she handed me the five-dollar bill she'd received from a family friend for her birthday. I bought the movie tickets, lunch at a diner near the theater, and popcorn and soda for Becky. Afterward, when we were waiting for the Handi-Van, Becky grew irritable and I asked what was wrong. Glaring at me, she said she wanted to know if I had used up that whole five dollars. I showed her a stub to indicate that her movie ticket alone had cost more than that, but she remained suspicious.

Staff members often took a group to lunch at a nearby diner, and I told them I'd learned that one day Becky had felt embarrassed when it was time to pay for her meal. Shortly afterward when I met Becky's Handi-Van for an appointment at Queen's Hospital, she greeted me by saying, "I'm angry with you; you didn't give me enough money for lunch!!" I explained that I had given her two five-dollar bills, which amounted to ten dollars. The lunch cost around seven dollars, more than enough for the meal, and she should have received about three dollars in change. Still indignant, she shouted: "You never told me that!"

Becky remained in this outpatient program for several years. When she was close to graduating, a social worker on staff asked me if she still wanted to live independently, and I said that Becky was understandably frustrated in her group homes, where her roommates were often women whose mental problems were worse than her own. But, I added, I felt that Becky had become more realistic about her limitations and no longer mentioned living on her own.

But Becky's fears surfaced as graduation loomed. She began a session with Joyce by complaining at length about other group home residents, but finally admitted that she'd been acting up because she was nervous about the future. She said to me, "I don't want to graduate because I got nothing to do afterwards, and I'll miss my friends."

My brother was in town and we went to the graduation ceremony, bringing leis for Becky. When she saw us she said, "Oh, no," but she was grinning. We reminded Becky that completing the program was a great accomplishment. Shortly after that, when Becky was about to be assigned a new social worker, her psychiatrist wrote this assessment:

> During the years when Ms. Rebecca Norris has been a patient at Kōkua Kalihi Valley, her emotional state has been a roller coaster. It was only in recent years that she has remained stable, except for minor ups and downs. Her medications were adjusted until she was maintained at her usual level of functioning.

In her first group home, where she lived for several years, her behavior was often unpredictable. She constantly complained to me about the other residents. But as she settled in, she became easier to live with. The caregiver learned her ways, and vice versa. She has had trouble adjusting to new group home placements but her family and especially her sister Kathy remain supportive of her. She takes her to the movies on weekends.

Miss Norris recently graduated from the Queen's Day Program. She looks forward to going back to Clubhouse. She talks about making new friends there. When seen today, she is well-groomed as usual and appears in good physical health. She walks unassisted and balances herself by walking with her feet slightly apart. As usual, she loves to talk and shares proudly about her graduation, and receiving leis from her brother and sister. She also proudly shows off the blue colored fingernails done by a friend. There is no sign of any major thought disorder like paranoia or delusion. Mood is euthymic. No self-injurious ideation is expressed. Except for hand tremors, no other EPS/TF is observed or reported.

"MANICKY"

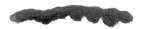

THE LANGUAGE PHYSICIANS EMPLOY to describe physical conditions is precise, but when they venture into psychology they're forced to resort to the language of poetry, their need to be accurate colliding with the tendency of words to remain stubbornly subjective and allusive.

Some descriptions of Becky provided by doctors are straightforward: "Patient is alert, verbally responsive. Coherent and organized. Not depressed." Others are more suggestive: "Affect: constricted." "Cognitive function: grossly intact." "Speech: pressured." I was glad to see Becky frequently referred to as a "fair historian," as I knew she kept herself well-informed about her medical problems.

When Becky went to extremes, the medical language also became extreme. "Mood incongruent, labile. Thought process: linear briefly with some flight of ideas, occasional derailment, occasional word salad." The term *word salad* is commonly used to describe the verbal communication of someone who is in the manic phase of bipolar disorder, but it's also a potent metaphor for artistic technique: the "word salad" of poetry.

Having been in conversation with two people who were in the midst of a psychotic episode triggered by severe pneumonia—my husband and my sister—I can tell you that it feels like being inside a surrealist poem. Both David and Becky were making sense, referring to real events and people, but in a disjointed and haphazard way that was difficult to follow if you didn't know them well. That may say more about my own thought processes than I want to admit, yet I wonder if "disjointed, haphazard speech" is a term the medical profession might find useful.

Once when a severe infection triggered delusions in Becky, I was surprised to find she had regressed so far that she was living in her troubled past. The emergency room physician's notes read: "She fears that she has gotten into legal trouble." He added, "Insight and judgment are rated poor. She's floridly delusional, saying 'We were all raped by the same person and I wonder if I am pregnant.' Mood extremely labile, mood swings from tearful to euphoria and giggling."

After consulting with a psychiatrist, the doctor admits Becky to a medical ward and puts her on IV antibiotics. By the second day she is much improved. The doctor writes that she's speaking of "trying to think happy thoughts, and says that everyone is beautiful in their own way. Still paranoid but consolable, and happy to hear that the police are not after her and that people are not trying to harm her." On the third day, she's well enough to be released and I take her to a movie.

On another occasion a physician trying to determine whether to admit Becky to a medical ward for a urinary tract infection or the psych ward noted that the "patient's psychosis and agitation continued despite medical evidence of improvement on antibiotics. EEG was obtained to differentiate delirium verses decompensated bipolar disorder." The doctor notes that she was also experiencing "intermittent agitation with poor hygiene—urinating on herself."

When this physician suggested to Becky that she be admitted to the hospital for her infection but also have consultations with a psychiatrist and counselor, she readily agreed. The notes read: "She accepted treatment plan. Somewhat disorganized. Complained of feeling 'manicky' with racing thoughts."

I was glad to find additional notes from Becky's Kōkua Valley internist, who added a prescription for physical therapy because "Becky deteriorates even over a short hospital stay." More importantly, she describes the Becky she knows, writing, "She has had acute delirium in the past whenever she gets an infection. Baseline mental status is quite pleasant and although she can be a little manic, she can carry on a cohesive conversation, has a good memory and attention to detail. However, when she gets an infection, she is unable to speak coherently, is tangential in her thought process with pressured speech."

It was crucial for Becky to have a physician who knew her and could insert valuable information into the medical file, giving anyone treating Becky a sense of who she was as a person. This doctor was able to speak for Becky at a time when she was unable to speak for herself.

But leave it to my sister to come up with the best term to describe her state: "manicky." Thank you, Becky. That's the word we've needed all along.

"I FEEL OK ABOUT HER GOING"

In the autumn of 2009, it became clear that our ninety-two-year-old mother was dying. One day at lunch she said, "Nothing tastes good anymore," and a few weeks later she was unable to lift a fork to feed herself. Her body was slowly shutting down, and John, Charlotte, and I decided to put her into home hospice. John and Marilyn came from the mainland and rented a car large enough to put Becky's wheel-chair in the trunk, making sure she had frequent visits with Mom, who was growing weaker by the day. Mom still knew us and responded to our presence with brilliant smiles.

On the last day of her life, Mom had difficulty even opening her eyes. We still got an occasional smile, and Mom responded with a faint squeeze if any of us took her hand. John went to get Becky, and she took Mom's hand and told her that she loved her. When I accompanied my brother in taking Becky back home, we told her Mom would not live much longer. Becky said she understood; later she told me that after we left she went to her room and cried.

Our mother slipped away early the next morning. I went to Becky's place and when she saw me she knew that Mom had died. That was on a Friday; by Sunday Becky wanted to go to a movie. She seemed all right, but we knew she'd have a difficult time with the memorial at Mom's senior living place and the funeral at my church. We made ar-rangements for Becky to have some quiet time by herself in my brother's hotel room between those events. In her journal Becky wrote that she had told Joyce, "I feel okay about mom going because I talked to her before she died."

Becky's birthday came a few weeks after Mom's death, and Charlotte and I held a celebration at a Chinese restaurant of Becky's choice in downtown Honolulu. Becky had a grand time being the center of attention and opening gifts. I gave her the usual cosmetics and a subscription to a fashion magazine, but I had also bought a stuffed panda that played a silly song that Becky liked. It made her laugh, and she played it over and over during our meal.

But Becky's grief took a toll. Having both parents gone is a new and uncomfortable feeling. You're orphaned, and sense that no one will ever love you with that unconditional love that your parents gave you. It proved too much for Becky to handle.

"I TELL THEM ALL ABOUT IT"

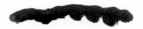

ONE OF BECKY'S HOSPITAL stays with pneumonia and a urinary tract infection occurred shortly after Becky had met a grandniece, the first member of our family's new generation. Becky had been excited when our niece became pregnant and had enjoyed looking at photos of the newborn baby. I was surprised that on first meeting the seventeen-month-old girl Becky had seemed distracted and was less talkative than usual. Our family reunions are increasingly rare, as people must now fly to Hawaii from the mainland, and I knew that Becky had been looking forward to seeing everyone.

I received a phone call from Becky's caregiver not long after we took her home. Becky had become increasingly agitated and did not want to take her medication. She became so manic that her caregiver had called 911. I was on my way to the emergency room again.

Becky's odd behavior was due in part to her infections. But I believe that psychological stress was also present, with Becky unconsciously regarding this child as an unwelcome reminder of the passage of time, and a significant change in the fabric of the family. Becky was now a member of our oldest generation.

After observing Becky's odd response to meeting her grandniece I wondered if she was especially troubled because the child had been born close to the one-year anniversary of our mother's death. Becky was a magical thinker, avid to find patterns in events and thread loose connections together. For her there were no coincidences, and I sensed that the recent juxtaposition of a death and a birth in the family had affected Becky in ways she couldn't control. Postpartum depression is common in women who've just given birth, but I began to wonder if Becky was suffering from a version of it that had less to do with physiology than with psychology.

I sent a note to Joyce, Becky's longtime counselor, saying that "while Becky is happy about this baby, her birth, combined with the deaths of our parents, is a big change. I think Becky doesn't know how to respond to her mixed feelings, other than to regress and act out."

Becky didn't understand that the anxiety she felt was normal. When she had recovered and was out of the hospital, I told her that I had also felt a strange mix of emotions when the baby was born. I had loved being an aunt, and now relished the thought of being a great-aunt. But I also felt a nagging sadness. I suggested to Becky that it might help to remember how thrilled our deceased parents would be to have a great-grandchild. Becky smiled. "Oh," she said, "I tell them all about it."

HOLY WEEK

BECKY DID NOT DISGUISE her mental illness. If we were dining out and a waiter asked if she wanted to start with a cocktail, she would reply, firmly, "No; it would interfere with my psych meds."

Medication kept Becky fairly stable, so it was easy to tell if something was wrong. And one day a cab driver we used regularly for our movie excursions, a man who had a brother with schizophrenia, phoned me to say he was concerned about Becky. When he had picked her up she was speaking rapidly, repeating herself in an increasingly agitated manner. I planned to take Becky to a movie that day, and after the driver dropped her off at the theater where we met, I became worried as well. This manic state was the worst I had seen in some time.

Becky was better during the movie, but occasionally she'd mutter to herself as if I weren't there. When the driver came to take Becky home, I decided to accompany her, and at the home I asked him to wait so I could talk with the caregiver. I told her that as Becky seemed exceptionally manic, I wanted her to keep me informed about her condition.

A few hours later, she phoned and said that Becky had gotten so out of control she'd called 911. When I arrived at the emergency room, the physician told me he'd noted that Becky had recently been treated for pneumonia, and as pneumonia often causes emotional disturbances, it was likely that her psychotropic medications needed to be readjusted. He had sent her to the hospital's psychiatric ward. When I went there and said that I wanted to see my sister, the staff was pleasant but firm: they wanted to assess Becky before allowing visitors.

The next morning a staff member phoned and said that Becky had been screaming, rolling on the floor, and biting her fingers. They had put her in a carpeted room and assigned her a medical sitter because she had tried to remove the Foley catheter that was draining urine from her bladder. She advised that I not visit that day but promised to keep in touch. It was Palm Sunday.

On Tuesday a nurse called and said that Becky had improved enough that I could visit. When I arrived I was shocked: Becky's appearance was a painful reminder of the time, many years before, when my husband had been diagnosed with "psychotic melancholia." We were then living in western South Dakota, and he'd been missing for three days. When the police in Bismarck, North Dakota, found him, they took him to a hospital. When I arrived a nurse directed me to the room where David had been placed. I entered, and seeing an old man hunched in a wheelchair, I almost walked out. Then I looked again. I hadn't recognized my husband, who looked as if he'd been turned inside out. He was forty-one years old. Becky, too, was barely recognizable: a fragile shell of herself, pale and in such emotional distress she couldn't look at me. All the bravado, the dynamic personality that normally sustained her had vanished, leaving a shadow of a person.

She spoke in a hoarse whisper, as if she'd been strangled and was struggling to regain her voice. One hand was swollen, bandaged where she had bitten herself and broken two fingers. Becky had no recollection of injuring herself. When visiting hours were over and I got ready to leave, she took my hand, looked me in the eye for the first time and asked if I could come again. Of course, I said. Tomorrow.

My Episcopal parish has evening services during much of Holy Week. On Monday night a Tenebrae service, on Tuesday singing hymns from Taizé, on Wednesday the Stations of the Cross, and on Thursday a service that commemorates when Jesus shared a meal with his disciples on the night before his death, instituting the Eucharist that the Christian church celebrates to this day. I missed all of it that year because the visiting hours at the psych ward were from seven to eight in the evening.

That's a difficult time for me, as I wake very early and by evening I'm ready for bed. But as I needed to be with my sister, I settled on a routine: I would walk or take a bus partway to the hospital every day in the fading light. After my visit, when it was dark and I was exhausted, I would take a taxicab home.

Becky improved slightly from night to night. By Wednesday she could look directly at me. By Thursday she could speak with a minimum of weeping. I told Becky I felt she was getting good care, and when I asked her if she felt safe, she said yes.

On Friday Becky was weepy again. She took my hand and told me she had something important to tell me. She said she'd had another visitor but didn't want anyone to know about him. She whispered, "He's my secret husband." I nodded, but was stunned, as seeking a stable relationship with a man had been such a long and fruitless struggle for her. But in her psyche she had found a husband who had visited her when she needed him most.

In the Hebrew Scriptures, the prophets often use the metaphor of husband and wife to describe God's relationship with humanity. Isaiah's chapter 54 is typical, stating, "Your Maker is your husband; the LORD of hosts is his name. . . . The LORD has called you like a wife forsaken and grieved in spirit" (Isaiah 54:5, 6). In the Christian tradition, the church is the bride of Christ. The term also refers to women in religious vows, who wear a wedding band. I was certain that Becky knew nothing of this, but in her raw need she'd tapped into a deep archetype. *Oh, Jesus Christ*, I thought, *you come when you are called.*

A nurse took me aside and asked if Becky had told me about the secret husband. Nearly in tears herself, she said, "Isn't that the saddest thing you've ever heard?" I replied that Becky's life had been exceptionally difficult, marked by a loneliness that even a loving family couldn't overcome. Not having a partner had troubled Becky more as our parents aged and died, and she entered middle age. I added that maybe it wasn't entirely sad that Becky had found a secret husband who gave her hope, one who could not be taken from her.

Becky was released from the hospital late on Holy Saturday. I took her home in a cab and slept for the rest of that day and most of Easter Sunday. I didn't worship with my parish at all that week; I had been attending an altogether different church. My sister never mentioned her secret husband again.

PART SEVEN

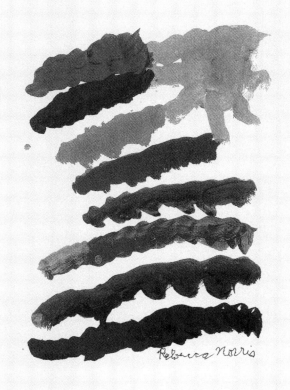

Rebecca Norris

"Here We Go Again"

"SHE'S A MOTHER HEN AND I'M FED UP WITH HER"

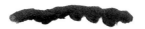

My feelings toward my sister ran the gamut: I loved her, and she exasperated me. I tried to do my best for Becky but knew that she would say that my record was spotty. Much of what I experienced with Becky would be recognizable to anyone who has a sister.

Becky didn't hesitate to lay out her frustrations with me in her sessions with Joyce. On one occasion, while it's clear that Becky is contending with a load of problems, it's me that she settles on as the one to blame. Joyce's notes read:

> Becky admits to being in a bad mood. She's fallen twice at home and has a bruised knee. She's in trouble with the group home operators because she stole $10.00 from them. She feels ashamed, and is working on a way to pay them back. She's been suspended from the Handi-Van because she cancelled so many rides at the last minute. She's feuding with two other residents of the home and says that she's trying to forgive them because of their illness. But isolating herself from them means that she can't watch television, and now she's spending too much time alone in her room, which she knows is not good for her. She says her main complaint is her sister Kathy. "She's a mother hen and I'm fed up with her."

If I seemed overbearing to Becky, it may have been because I was trying to make up for lost time. I was now the family member closest at hand, and that meant that I came face to face with all of Becky's moods and emotions. There were times when she said mean things intending to hurt me, and other times when she clearly needed consolation and reassurance. I learned to navigate through the storms and calms.

In one session with Joyce, Becky complained that going to the movies with me had become the only time all week she left the house. Her caregiver asked me to inform her but not tell Becky when I'd be taking her out, as she'd become so excited the night before that she'd wet her bed. It was a blessing to take Becky to the movies, an obligation but also a joy. I couldn't make up for all the years we'd spent apart, but I could enjoy getting to know Becky better.

"I WISH I COULD BE LIKE HIM"

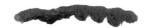

TO MY SISTER, A MOVIE MEANT getting away from her group home for a few hours and being treated to lunch, a soda, and popcorn. From her point of view, there could be no such thing as a bad movie. For years my goal in life was to find a movie that Becky would like and I could stand. She didn't like slasher or horror films, but everything else was fair game.

Years of sitting through dreadful movies with my sister has convinced me that this is one thing Jesus had in mind when he exhorted his disciples to go the extra mile. It's also proof that asceticism finds you where you are, and it can mean sitting through a so-called romantic, so-called comedy without complaint.

In choosing movies I followed Becky's lead. She considered animated films childish. Batman and Spider-Man didn't interest her, but she liked Superman and Iron Man. Often as we watched a preview for a film that seemed especially awful, she would say, "That looks good," and I groaned inwardly. When I told her that *Sex and the City* had opened and asked if she'd like to see it, to my relief she responded with an indignant "No!"

Becky displayed little interest in the technology of filmmaking, but once she asked, "How do they make it rain?" She had realized that filmmakers were manipulating the rainy scenes and was amused if a bit disbelieving when I told her that large overhead sprinklers are commonly used.

One day Becky asked, "How do they make people look dead?" I responded by making a "dead face." Becky responded in kind, and we held a "dead face" showdown over lunch. I told her that filmmakers often made plastic replicas of actors' faces, and even whole bodies. Becky found this gross.

My sister's reactions to a movie could surprise me. When I asked her how she liked 2009's hyperactive *Sherlock Holmes*, Becky said, "It made me sad." She explained that the carriages, horses, and period clothing had reminded her of our mother's parents, long deceased. "When I saw those old things I thought of them," Becky said, "and it made me want to cry." I was curious to know what she thought of Sherlock Holmes himself. She said, "Oh, I like him. He figures everything out. I wish I could be like him."

Some decisions about movies for Becky were easy to make. Films with subtitles were out, as the words came and went too fast for her. But it was difficult for me to tell what my sister could tolerate in terms of complexity. When I took Becky to see *The Life of Pi*, I told her that the story might not make sense, but that the visual imagery was supposed to be beautiful. We both loved the sight of the whale emerging from the ocean at night, aglow with phosphorescence, but as we were leaving the theater Becky complained that she didn't understand the movie. I told her that I didn't know what to make of it either, so maybe she should ask herself the question that comes at the end: Which story do you prefer, the one with the tiger, or the one without? Becky grinned and said, "The one with the tiger!" I replied, "Me, too. And maybe that's enough."

Another movie that Becky liked but found somewhat confusing is the little-known but rewarding *Moon* with Sam Rockwell. I had gone alone to see it and decided that my sister would enjoy the movie, as she'd resonate with the film's theme of loneliness. Rockwell plays a man who monitors a mechanized mining operation on the moon. His only contacts with other people come in videophone conversations with his wife and young daughter on earth.

The plot reveals itself slowly, and I had warned Becky that in this film many things were not as they seemed. Suspecting that she would enjoy the challenge, I said that if she paid close attention, I thought she'd be able to figure everything out. Becky watched intently and whispered an occasional question. I told her to keep watching. She was puzzled by the relationship of the man with his family back home but quick to comprehend that he was being deceived by the mining corporation in an exceptionally cruel way.

This is a rare science fiction film with enough heart to make a person cry. My sister and I both lost it when Rockwell's character looks wistfully at the earth and says, "I want to go home."

WHAT I OWE TO
JOSEPH GORDON-LEVITT

I HAVE JOSEPH GORDON-LEVITT to thank for one of the best conversations I ever had with my sister. He's an actor I've admired ever since I saw his work in *Mysterious Skin*, about the aftereffects of childhood sex abuse on two young men. A new film he was starring in, *The Lookout*, sounded like a film Becky would like, but I had second thoughts about taking a person who had brain damage to a movie about a young man with brain damage. I knew Becky had seen *Rain Man* with Mom and Dad on its release in 1988 and wrote to me that "I wish more people would see it so they would understand me better." Becky did not have autism, but she clearly identified with a character who struggled to be appreciated and understood by other people. I told Becky a little about *The Lookout* and said that if it made her uncomfortable and she wanted to leave, we'd find another film at the multiplex.

I was not prepared for the way she took to the film, so much so that she asked if we could see it a second time. Becky had taken some of the classes depicted in the movie that help people with brain damage, such as learning how to sequence. Sequencing becomes important in *The Lookout*, as the young man uses it against the criminals who've assumed that because he's suffered brain damage, they can take advantage of him. They regard him as an easy and disposable mark, but he proves them wrong.

After we'd sat through the movie—twice—I asked my sister about the sequencing classes she had taken. Remembering them triggered some good memories, a time in her life when she had been successful at learning new things. I commented that the character in the film had been a lot smarter than people gave him credit for and that I'd always felt this was true of her. Becky nodded and rolled her eyes. "But"—I said—"you've been able to outsmart them, right? Like the guy in the movie?" She said, "You better believe it!"

A few years later I was visiting New York City when I noticed an ad for a new film, *Uncertainty*, starring Joseph Gordon-Levitt, that was being premiered at the IFC Center. The director and actors would be on hand for a discussion after the screening. I went, and at the theater was startled to see Joseph Gordon-Levitt, looking all of sixteen years old, sitting—or more accurately, fidgeting—in a seat across the aisle.

I enjoyed the film, as its scenery brought back memories: China-town, the first neighborhood I lived in when I came to the city after graduating from college, and Brooklyn, where I had worked in the early 1970s to provide poetry readings in public parks and libraries. At the discussion following the movie I bided my time, but as the questions dwindled I spoke up.

I thanked Gordon-Levitt for his work in *The Lookout*. I explained that as my sister was living with brain damage, I'd been apprehensive about taking her to see it, but she loved it. I added that while I take her to many films, I felt that this was the first time that she'd ever been able to fully identify with a character in a movie. It was the restraint and wisdom of his performance that had allowed her that. He replied with a "Thanks" and then an "Oh, wow," as the import of what I had said sank in. He commented that out of all his movies, this was the one where he had done the most research. I said, "It shows, and I thank you." Then we all dispersed into the Manhattan night.

"A FREAK IN THIS WORLD"

OVER THE YEARS I had learned that when Becky had a physical illness, it manifested first in psychological symptoms. If she was growing increasingly manic, it usually meant that she had an infection.

I learned to listen closely to Becky whenever she was being treated in an emergency room. Once when she'd been diagnosed with pneumonia and we were waiting for her to be admitted to the hospital, I was surprised to hear her ranting about the past. She was bringing up names I hadn't heard in years. One was a former boyfriend who had treated her badly. Another was a roommate with whom she'd had a long-standing feud. This woman had bullied Becky, trying to talk her into giving her money and belongings, even gifts from the family, and reacted aggressively if Becky stood her ground.

To be fair, Becky could make life difficult for her roommates. If she felt that there wasn't enough drama in her life, she'd invent it. Once at a counseling session Becky had asked me to attend, I said I'd observed that in each of her group homes Becky would designate one person as her enemy. The family would then hear an ongoing stream of complaints about this person until either they or Becky moved out of the home. Then we'd start hearing complaints about someone new. Becky looked stunned and said, "I never thought about that." The counselor jumped in with, "That's why we're here; we can talk about it." And this is how, inch by inch, over the years, Becky progressed to adulthood.

But in that emergency room I was witnessing angry behavior I hadn't seen in over twenty years. Unlike in the past, however, Becky was self-aware enough to be distressed. Weeping, she said, "It's the old Becky; she's back." I replied, "But we know the new Becky is in there; we just have to find her."

Her treatment for pneumonia was successful and included a consultation with a psychiatrist that Becky said was helpful. Another thing that lifted Becky's spirits was an unexpected visit from her former caregiver, Mrs. R. Becky had moved out of her group home many years before. The next day, when I entered Becky's hospital room, she said, proudly, "You'll never guess who came to see me!"

A few days after Becky returned home, I asked if she'd like to celebrate her release from the hospital with lunch and a movie. She picked a film and said she'd look forward to "real food" again. But in the diner she suddenly burst into tears and said, "I feel like a freak in this world." She began reminiscing about the days when she'd been more independent, able to take the city bus on her own.

I asked Becky if she would like to try going several days a week to a daycare program. She said yes, and with the help of her social worker I found a good place. But Becky fretted about how she would get there, and if she had the right clothes. I told her we would work all that out, and if Medicaid didn't cover the cost, John and I would pay for it.

The staff was welcoming and sensitive to Becky's needs, offering her a number of activities. But as usual, Becky didn't fit in. Everyone there was at least twenty years older, and what was meant to assuage her loneliness only made her feel more alone. Her social worker recommended that she return to her former day program, the Clubhouse, where there were more people her own age.

Becky's social worker had recently retired and Becky's new advocate proved to be a blessing. She was young, still working on her master's degree in social work, and eager to help. I'll call her Carol. When she showed me the records she'd been given on Becky, I was shocked to discover no mention of the perinatal hypoxia that had caused my sister's brain damage. That information, so vital in understanding my sister, had been lost over the years. Carol was appalled and told me that having this medical diagnosis in Becky's records would have made a difference, making it clear that physical damage was the root cause of much of Becky's mental instability and distress.

I found other errors and was glad to correct them. Becky had been described as a "dishwasher" who was "born and raised in Maryland." Becky moved with the family to Honolulu when she was seven, and while she had a complicated work history, she'd spent more time as an aide to disabled children than as a dishwasher. I wondered if her previous social worker couldn't believe Becky was capable of anything more than menial work and hadn't bothered to check.

Becky liked Carol, but didn't make things easy for Carol or me. Fortunately her attempts to manipulate us were transparent enough that we could counter them. Becky had told me that Clubhouse wouldn't let her return if she was using a walker or wheelchair, and told Carol that a doctor had put her on a new medication and recommended that she stay at home. Both were lies. Carol knew that Clubhouse wanted Becky to return, and I knew that Becky had not recently had a change in her medication. In talking with Carol, I said that I hoped that once Becky realized we were comparing notes she might learn not to lie to us.

I told Carol that when Becky had been placed in a nursing home to recover after one of her hospitalizations for pneumonia, she had thrived there. In its structured environment her gregarious personality flourished and she approached every activity with gusto, making potholders, playing bingo, watching Korean soap operas, and attending every worship service—Protestant, Catholic, Buddhist.

I'd been frustrated when I was told that an assessment showed that while Becky needed substantial help with daily tasks such as bathing and dressing, her condition did not yet merit nursing home care. As Becky was now becoming more physically frail, I asked Carol if we could get a new assessment; it revealed that while Becky still couldn't be placed in a nursing home, she now qualified for an intermediate step, an adult foster care program. Carol agreed to find a placement for Becky in a home with fewer residents and more medical services.

"I LIKE IT HERE"

FOR BECKY'S PHYSICAL NEEDS, her new living situation made sense. But the move was devastating for her psychological health. My biggest regret is that I failed to recognize what would happen when Becky suddenly lost both the friction and the vital human connections that group homes had provided.

She had gone from the lively if often stressful environment of a group home to a place where the only other resident was a woman in her nineties who was bedridden and unable to speak. My sociable, extroverted sister was alone for much of the time. I could resolve to take her out more often, and fortunately her new caregivers, unlike her previous ones, included Becky in their frequent family gatherings. Becky enjoyed gossiping with the adult children and playing with young grandchildren.

I enrolled Becky in a variety of adult day programs, but none lasted long. As the outpatient psychiatric program at Queen's Hospital had been an excellent place for Becky, I asked if she might return there but was told that it wasn't possible. Clubhouse no longer worked for her either.

I suspect that Becky's loneliness made the diagnosis of esophageal cancer she received—ten years after her breast cancer—feel like liberation, as treatments would get her out of the house, and she'd have daily contact with the staff at the Queen's Cancer Center. After our first visit Becky said, "I like it here."

I liked it there as well. Being in waiting rooms at oncology treatment centers with my husband had taught me that while many people there are clearly struggling with the dire effects of treatment, these places are not necessarily depressing. You witness many acts of love: a large man holding his wife's purse for her as he gently guides her through the clinic doors, a young woman clasping her husband's hand and allowing him to rest his head on her shoulder.

As Becky began her weekly visits for treatment, I devised instructions for "How to Run a Cancer Center":

- On a patient's second visit, when the person is being wheeled to the desk to sign in, have the receptionist look up, smile, and say, "It's OK, Becky. We know you're here."

- Offer a free weekly art class taught by a former oncology nurse who is herself a cancer survivor.

- Have a therapy dog, preferably a golden lab named Yoda. And when a patient shows up on a day between appointments and says "I'm feeling a little down, and would like to see Yoda," have the dog come out with a nurse and allow the patient to pet the dog and give him a treat.

"HERE WE GO AGAIN"

AN EMERGENCY ROOM PHYSICIAN once explained to me that Becky's recurring pneumonia was likely caused by gastrointestinal reflux. Becky had been diagnosed with GERD, a reflux disease, and Barrett's esophagus, a precancerous condition. Becky's voice contained a note of satisfaction as she told the family about this diagnosis and new dietary restrictions that had been placed on her. She explained that her caregivers had placed a shim under the head of her bed to elevate it, and the doctor had told her to be careful not to lie down too soon after eating.

Becky bragged about being one of the first patients in Hawaii to receive the HALO ablation therapy for Barrett's. Her gastroenterologist said that while many patients suffer severe pain with this treatment, Becky had tolerated it well. Sadly, delays in Becky's treatment schedule caused by her caregivers added to her risk. Few people with GERD develop Barrett's esophagus, but Becky did. Few people with Barrett's develop cancer, but Becky did.

I was with Becky when she received the diagnosis of esophageal cancer. She rolled her eyes and said to the oncologist, "Here we go again." He told us that radical surgery was the only cure; it involved removing the cancerous section of the esophagus and reconnecting it with the stomach. "Other treatments might work," he said, "but this is the only cure." He seemed puzzled when we said we wanted to ask a surgeon if this operation would be right for Becky. He repeated, "But it's the only cure."

Becky and I worked on a list of questions for the surgeon. We wanted to know about potential complications as well as recovery time. When we met with him, he said that two major incisions were required, one in the chest, and one lower in the abdomen, and when we mentioned Becky's previous hernia surgery, he said that scar tissue would make the new operation more difficult. After Becky told him that she sometimes "went a little psycho" after surgery, he recommended that she not have the operation, as it had triggered severe psychological effects in several of his patients. He added that even if she tolerated the surgery, recovery would be long and difficult; Becky would be risking a drastic loss of her already limited mobility. But, he added, the decision was up to her. God bless her, Becky said she'd take her chances with radiation and chemotherapy. And God bless that honest and compassionate surgeon.

I was sad but also relieved. My main concern had been about Becky's quality of life. She was agreeing to treatments that might not save her life, but she was choosing to have the best possible life in whatever time she had left.

At her initial consultation with the oncologist who would be providing her treatments, Becky told him about hearing voices. She said, "I hear them in my head, and they say bad things to me. But I don't listen to them. Sometimes they want me to hurt myself, but I won't do it."

The doctor suggested that Becky be treated at the Queen's Cancer Center. If Becky began to show psychological distress, he could easily put her in the psych ward with no interruption in her treatment. Becky knew the psych ward staff had helped her in the past and said, "That's a good idea."

Becky came through her treatment in good spirits. She did not return to the psych ward.

"THE DIVINE PRESENCE IS EVERYWHERE"

SAINT BENEDICT IN HIS RULE OF LIFE for monks states, "We believe that the divine presence is everywhere" (ch. 19, v. 1). I became a Benedictine oblate in 1987, but Becky never asked me what that meant. And at the time I wouldn't have known what to tell her; I was slow to grasp how being an oblate would change my life. But by the time Becky's cancer treatments meant that we spent a lot of time at Queen's Hospital, I'd become convinced that God indeed is everywhere. And I could accept what caring for Becky meant, even when I had to turn down an invitation for a luncheon with Archbishop Desmond Tutu, who was visiting Episcopal churches in Hawaii. The date conflicted with an important consultation at the cancer center and accompanying Becky took precedence.

Sometimes appreciating God's presence meant transforming duty into fun. Becky liked that I had to work hard to push her wheelchair up the hospital's many ramps. The long climb from the dining room to the cancer center was especially challenging, and one day Becky asked if it would help if she yelled, "Cowabunga!" as I pushed. I told her it couldn't hurt.

We had long waits for Becky's Handi-Vans every day, but as we waited we took advantage of the people-watching that a hospital provides. We enjoyed seeing young couples leave with their newborn babies, and once witnessed a dazed-looking pair taking twins home.

We encountered friends from church or people who'd been fans of our dad's band. I'd see a high school classmate, or Becky might spot a former roommate. We conversed about movies or the family, and I would use my phone to show her new photos of our grandnieces. By this time there were two.

Watching a stream of white sedans, we took pleasure in the appearance of oddballs like an old silver Mercedes sedan, a woodie station wagon, a sleek black sports car paired with fiery stripes, florists' vans with paintings of bouquets, and courtesy vans from car dealerships whose sides depicted ocean waves, palm trees, and surfers. When you pay attention, you find more than you expect.

When you pay attention, you can find much more than just a way to pass the time. You can turn any place into holy ground. I had learned years before, when I was caregiving for my husband, that no matter how mundane my chores, the time we spent together was invaluable. Once he was gone, I would have memories that no one could take from me.

People are sometimes surprised to find that Benedictine men and women don't talk a lot about Jesus. This is part of their tradition; the monks of the fourth century often warn that talking about religion can lead to arguments and foster spiritual pride. It is said of Abba Poemen that when a renowned church official came to him and "began to speak of the Scriptures, and of spiritual things," the abba turned his face away and did not respond. The man, dismayed, prepared to leave, and monks asked Poemen to explain his behavior. He replied that this man "is great, and speaks of heavenly things and I am lowly and speak of earthly things. If he had spoken of the passions of the soul, I should have replied, but he speaks of spiritual things and I know nothing about that." On hearing this the visitor returned and asked Poemen, "What should I do, Abba, for the passions of the soul master me?" The elder then was happy to engage in conversation with him.

My sister's spirituality exemplified this down-to-earth approach. She certainly harbored an understanding of hospitality as expressed in chapter 53 of Benedict's Rule, which states that "all guests who present themselves are to be welcomed as Christ." At the hospital she was determined to learn the names of all the parking lot attendants, and several began giving her hugs every day.

Becky was doing her best to live with cancer, and the least I could do was help. She wasn't familiar with Saint Benedict's admonition, "Day by day remind yourself that you are going to die"; I suspect she would have found it morbid. But she knew she was in danger of dying and that made her all the more open to loving others. And I knew that being with Becky, waiting an hour each day for her Handi-Van, was the best possible use of my time.

DAISY

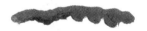

BECKY LOVED THE FASHION magazines I gave her. She would often hand me pages she'd torn out with photos of designer clothing that attracted her, so that I could search for similar items at discount stores.

Becky loved cosmetics because they allowed her to express her personality through color. One Christmas a niece gave her a set of nail polishes, and Becky painted each nail, a bit sloppily, in a different color and showed them off to the nurses at the cancer center.

When Becky became enamored of Daisy, a Marc Jacobs perfume, I worried that it might have an exorbitant price. But for twenty-five dollars I found a roll-on stick that would be easier for Becky to handle than a spray.

Becky wore Daisy during her cancer treatments, and now if I catch its scent, I see her entering the reception area as cheerfully as if she were arriving at a party. She'd ask the receptionists and nurses if they'd had a good weekend and how their children were doing. This place had become the center of Becky's social life, and she took this to mean that she had a duty to care for the people who worked there.

After her initial radiation and chemo ended, she took construction paper and crayons and made thank-you cards for the doctor, nurses, and receptionists. For the three-month checkup after her chemotherapy ended, Becky made a Christmas card for her oncologist. She explained that although it was only October, she wouldn't be seeing him until the next checkup in February.

As he looked at Becky's drawings of Santa and a decorated tree and tried to read the words she'd written so clumsily, he looked so startled that I realized that while he had understood from the outset that Becky had special needs, he had never before encountered such stark evidence of her brain damage. Her drawings must have looked to him like those of his four-year-old son.

Becky also gave two cards to a nurse, one for her and one for her five-year-old daughter. She explained that she didn't want the child to be jealous when she saw her mother's card.

THE COLOR ARTIST

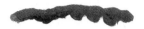

THE FAMILY HAD LONG KNOWN that Becky loved to draw and paint. For her birthdays and at Christmas we provided art supplies—drawing and construction paper, pastels and crayons thick enough for her to manipulate easily.

On our first visit to the Queen's Cancer Center I had noticed a poster advertising a free art class for cancer patients, their families, and caregivers. On obtaining the details at the reception desk, I told Becky that it met twice a week at the center, and we could easily adapt her schedule so she could attend.

At the first session, the teacher welcomed us and said that the project she'd planned that day was painting a flower pot. I produced a pot with puny-looking flowers, but Becky covered her pot inside and out with bold streaks of color. The teacher told her, "You're a natural colorist," and Becky beamed. She thought the teacher had said, "You're a color artist." Becky worked quickly, and when she was finished with the pot, the teacher provided her with paper and paint. Becky created a stunning abstract rainbow, signed it, and gave it to the teacher as a gift. It is also the art used on the cover and throughout this book.

This was the beginning of an important friendship for Becky. She told me she appreciated this teacher because she always made her feel included. When the project required fine motor skills Becky lacked, the teacher would give her materials so she could paint pictures. Becky said that in the past, when she couldn't do an assignment for a class, she was simply left out.

This had been the case when Becky was in elementary school and received failing grades in art. Her natural gifts had gone unnoticed, probably because ill-trained teachers couldn't imagine that a "slow" student could be creative. Now Becky flourished, and her teacher called her fearless for being willing to work in new mediums. At each class Becky painted feverishly, with torrents of color: a fan palm under a turbulent sky of gold and dark green, the green of the Koolau Mountains awash in rain, a rough landscape of brown earth with a fierce orange sky, and a lone traveler standing on the banks of a wide river. She occasionally painted pictures of delicate flowers in soft colors and asked me to send one to a grandniece. There were now three, and Becky wanted each of them to have some of her art.

Hawaii's Queen Emma, who founded the hospital in 1859, had an interest in botany, and to beautify the grounds she imported rare plants and trees from Asia. I had never heard of the Bombax tree until the teacher brought some of its blossoms to the class, hoping to inspire the students. Although Becky was not feeling well that day, she laughed when she saw the flower; it looked like a party favor that had exploded. Its silky pink tassels were surrounded by pink, satin-like curls, and Becky happily spent the class hour painting them.

Along with the making of art, these classes provided a respite from treatments and an opportunity for cancer patients to talk about their lives. When I showed Father Michael the work Becky was doing, he framed her work and arranged for it to be displayed in the church's parish hall. Becky was pleased that several people from the art class came to see the exhibit, and many people from the church complimented her on her work.

"THANK YOU FOR TELLING ME"

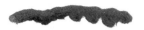

BECKY'S NEWFOUND CAPACITY for gratitude was a wonderment. For many years Becky's first response to anything you tried to tell her was an exasperated, "I know!" It was difficult to offer correction and impossible to warn Becky that she'd misconstrued a situation in a way that could have unfortunate consequences. She'd go into full defensive mode, stiffening her body and clenching her fists. Her eyes would narrow as if she was daring you to say anything more so she could go on the attack.

The change began when Becky was in her fifties and enrolled in an outpatient psychiatric program at Queen's. The staff had convinced Becky that people who corrected her were not necessarily disrespecting her; they might be doing her a favor. And Becky became a true believer. The family began hearing, "Thank you for telling me," as Becky's stock response to anyone who told her something she didn't know.

Her thanks were sincere. Becky was grateful that others were willing to help her. Her face softened and her body relaxed as she laid her weapons down.

PART EIGHT

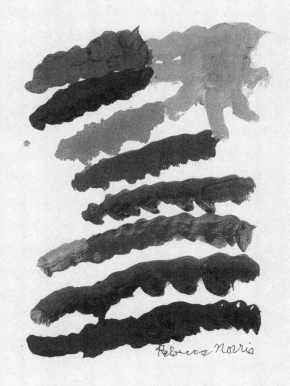

Rebecca Norris

"I Bet I Can Have Dessert Now"

"I'M AFRAID THAT
I'LL DIE ALONE"

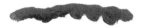

FROM THE TIME BECKY was very young, family parties and holiday celebrations engendered tears. She felt there was something wrong with her, but we told her it was all right if she needed time alone, and we got used to hearing loud "conversations" coming from Becky's room, as she talked to herself, trying to convince herself that she could rejoin us as we enjoyed a birthday cake or opened presents. Christmas, especially, was a difficult time.

One year I convinced her to come with me for Christmas Eve services at a church near her group home. At Kaumakapili, a historic church with many native Hawaiian members, I suspected that the service would be low-key, and Becky would be comfortable wearing a muumuu and slippers. At one church she had attended with Mrs. R., she had felt out of place because the women there wore fancier clothes than anything she owned.

The service ended with the congregation standing in a circle on the lawn. Blessed by a light rainfall, we sang "Silent Night" in Hawaiian and English. Becky began to weep and said she felt embarrassed. I told her that it was okay to cry in church, that I sometimes cry in church, and that church is a good place to let the tears come. I said that people in the earliest Christian churches had called tears a gift from God. She seemed surprised to hear this, but looked relieved.

In Becky's last years she attended Sunday services with me at St. Clement's, an Episcopal church in my neighborhood. She liked the people and enjoyed singing hymns in a loud voice with uncertain pitch. Some of the ritual was confusing to her, but she relaxed as she began to memorize some of the prayers and responses. She asked Father Michael to explain why people made the sign of the cross, and they practiced doing it together.

I would make Becky's Handi-Van reservations and meet her before the service, and also make sure she left the parish hall afterward in time to catch her ride home. Eventually Becky became bold enough to attend church when I was out of town. She knew people would look after her when she arrived—by this time she needed to be wheeled up a ramp into the sanctuary. Becky liked to arrive early enough to join the book discussion group. She'd listen intently but rarely spoke. Once when the priest asked Becky if she wanted to say something, she quickly responded with a slightly affronted, "No! I'm thinking!"

Our mother's funeral was held at St. Clement's, and my brother was inspired to ask Becky to carry Mom's ashes in her lap as she was wheeled to the front of the church. Becky solemnly handed the box of woven lauhala containing the ashes to the priest, who placed them on a small table that held a photograph of our mother that was draped with a lei. As I got up to give a eulogy, Becky tugged at my skirt and muttered, "Don't mess this up!" After the funeral, when I asked her how I had done, Becky shrugged and said, "You were okay."

One year I asked Becky if she'd like to stay with me over Christmas. We could attend the early Christmas Eve service at St. Clement's and then go to my apartment to watch movies. I'd give her my bed and sleep on the living room sofa. Becky enthusiastically agreed, and I got busy with preparations, stocking my refrigerator with Diet Coke and asking her caregivers to provide Becky's medications and loan me an incontinence pad for the bed.

At the church service, Becky enjoyed watching the children, but as we sang the familiar carols she began to weep. When I asked her what was troubling her, she said, "I'm afraid that I'll die alone, and there will be no one to take care of me." I hugged her and asked her if she'd like to talk to the priest after the service. She nodded and soon was singing again.

I will always be grateful to the priest for the way she comforted Becky that night. When Becky confided her fears in a hoarse whisper, the priest said, "Becky, you have too many people who care too much about you to ever abandon you." That was our Christmas blessing.

Becky had asked if I could order a pizza for dinner, a rare treat for her. I knew she enjoyed slapstick so I rented *A Night at the Opera*, and for romance, *Love, Actually*. I had no idea that it was a Christmas movie. Becky loved both films.

The next day, at Charlotte's house, Becky was cheerful again, gleefully opening her presents, glad that we had given her all the things on her wish list.

"I BET I CAN HAVE
DESSERT NOW"

BECKY'S ESOPHAGEAL CANCER had been designated as stage I-B, but experience with my husband had taught me not to put too much stock in that assessment. If you want evidence that medicine is much more an art than a hard science, spend some time with an oncologist.

Becky had been happy to learn that her new chemotherapy treatment would not cause hair loss. But the nurse warned that she might feel more susceptible to cold, and a cap could keep her head warm. When she opened a cabinet full of caps that volunteers had knit for the cancer center, Becky gasped. Pleased to be asked to choose one, she took her time and opted for one in blue and lavender. She asked me to take a photo with my phone so that the family could see her wearing it.

Eventually Becky had a port installed with a twenty-four-hour drip, and she liked to show off the little black bag she wore that contained the medication. We went to the cancer center every Saturday to have the port flushed and new medication installed; then we would go to a movie. Becky endured her treatment better than anyone had expected. We'd been told that people often lose weight during treatment, but in February, when we went for her next checkup, we learned that Becky had gained more than five pounds. I reminded her that a visit with her regular internist was coming in a few days, and she'd not be happy to see Becky gaining weight. Years before, this doctor had helped Becky improve her diet and get more exercise when obesity had added to her medical problems.

We had planned to go to lunch that day at Becky's favorite diner. But after she was weighed, I commented that she might not be able to have dessert. "Yes, sister!" Becky snapped at me, rolling her eyes. The nurse taking her vital signs laughed. "Sisters!" I said, and we all laughed. We were expecting the same good news we'd received at the consultation in October. But now the oncologist told us that to his surprise, Becky's cancer had returned with a vengeance. It had spread and was no longer treatable. "We can manage symptoms and pain," he said, "but that's it."

I was speechless, but Becky turned to me and said, "I bet I can have dessert now, can't I?" "Oh, yes," I replied, "as much dessert as you like." The doctor looked surprised, but I was glad to hear Becky being very much herself, even after receiving such devastating news. The doctor wanted to be certain that Becky understood the gravity of her situation, and when he asked if we wanted a prognosis, she looked at him suspiciously and asked, "What's that?" Growing up in our family Becky had acquired a large vocabulary, but this was a word she didn't know. When the oncologist explained that it meant he'd estimate how much longer she had to live, she said, "No way!"

I've never been more proud of my sister. I told her I thought that this was a wise decision; without a prognosis, she could go on living her life without worrying about when it would end. Becky said, "I think this will hit me later," and the doctor reminded her that she could always call the cancer center, and if she had any pain they could help. I said I'd explain the new situation to her caregiver and ask her to always let her use the phone if she wanted to call the doctor or me.

At lunch Becky ordered her favorite dish, spaghetti, and made her usual joke about her lifelong inability to pronounce the word, which came out as "pasketti." For dessert, she wanted red velvet cake with vanilla ice cream. I asked the waiter to bring the biggest piece of cake they had.

A few days later when we went to Kōkua Kalihi Valley, her doctor had received the report from the cancer center. She discussed our options for palliative care and hospice, and told Becky that the best prescription she could give was for her to have all the red velvet cake she wanted. Grinning broadly, Becky said, "You're a good doctor."

"DOES SHE HAVE FAITH?"

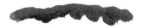

I HAD LEARNED FROM CAREGIVING for my husband that it was important for me not to ignore my own health. Fortunately we shared an internist who knew our situation and kept after me if I allowed myself to become so exhausted that I became ill. She knew that a year before my husband died in 2003, I had lost my father to aplastic anemia, and more recently I'd had difficulty coping after my mother's death.

In 2009 when I saw my doctor soon after my mother died, she said she felt I was suffering from a version of post-traumatic stress syndrome. I said that I didn't feel that I needed medication; just talking things out with her was help enough.

But now I told her I wanted combat pay, as I was again being plunged into caregiving for someone who was about to die. When I told the doctor a little about Becky's history, she asked, "Does she have faith?" No one had asked me that, not directly, and certainly not a physician who had been raised in Japan and with whom I had never discussed religion. For all I knew she was Buddhist or Shinto.

I hesitated but finally said, "Yes, my sister is a woman of faith, but she doesn't talk about it. I'd say that her faith is childlike, and solid. She likes going to church with me, she likes singing hymns, and she believes that angels are looking out for her." I had given Becky a small icon of the Archangel Michael that she carried in her backpack; she often told me that he had protected her from accidents.

I added, "I'm sure Becky believes that when she dies she'll be re-united with our parents and our grandparents, with all the people who have ever loved her."

"Good," the doctor said. "That should help."

I found her comment reassuring. Becky's belief that her death would bring the joy of reuniting with long-lost loved ones is a conviction shared by many people from a variety of religious traditions. But the doctor's question, coming out of the blue, had jolted me, and I thought again of Mary of Egypt and scholar Benedicta Ward's insight into the meaning of her story for us. She calls Mary "the sinful woman who receives the simple gift of salvation from Christ without any acts . . . sacraments or prayers, but only because of her great need." Mary of Egypt allows me to see my sister's "secret husband" in a new light. He surely accompanied her during the last great trial of her life.

Rebecca Sue Norris
Medications as of April 2013

DAILY:
Levothyroxine: 50 mcg by mouth
Depakote: 250 mg, 3 tablets by mouth twice a day
Protonix: 40 mg by mouth
Docusate Sodium: 100 mg by mouth twice a day (hold for loose BM)
Lovastatin: 10 mg by mouth
Seroquel: 100 mg by mouth three times a day (with meals)
Seroquel: 400 mg by mouth at bedtime
Travatan Eye Drops 0.0004%: 1 drop in each eye at bedtime
Benztropine: 0.5 mg by mouth twice a day
Multivitamin
Vitamin B12: 1000 mcg by mouth
Calcium Carbonate: 648 mg, 2 tablets by mouth three times a day
Ferrous Sulfate: 325 mg by mouth twice a day
Vitamin D: 400 IU, 1 tablet by mouth

WEEKLY:
Alendronate sodium: 70 mg by mouth every Sunday

AS NEEDED:
Hydrocortisone cream 2.5%: to rash as needed twice a day
Naphcon eye drops: 1 drop in each eye every 6 hours as needed for red eyes
Mylanta: 1 tablespoon by mouth every 6 hours as needed for indigestion
Seroquel: 100 mg by mouth as needed for agitation
Tylenol

ALLERGIES: Cogentin; penicillin; adhesive bandage tape

This list suggests to me that my sister was overmedicated. Mom and Dad had taken Becky off Mellaril when she was a teenager but generally trusted doctors when they prescribed new medications. From the 1960s on, as new psychotropic drugs came on the market, doctors were eager to try them. These medications have helped many people struggling with mental illness, but I can't shake the feeling that they've also been guinea pigs for any new drug that came along. I'm convinced that Becky's use of so many psychotropic medications over the years shortened her life.

"WE LEARN A LOT ABOUT LOVE"

WHEN BECKY FIRST SHOWED signs of the bipolar condition that would cause such distress to her and the family, Dad wrote in one of the Christmas letters he sent to family and friends, "We learn a lot about love from her."

On the day my sister was diagnosed with terminal cancer, I was angry. Becky'd had a hard time coming into this world, and now she'd have a hard time leaving it. I was angry at God, at the world, at everyone and everything. I mustered a little gratitude: that I'd been with her when she received the diagnosis, and that she'd enjoyed that red velvet cake. But I was angry.

When I arrived home from the cancer center, I was greeted by the sight of two brilliant rainbows stretching over my neighborhood into nearby Mānoa Valley, where the family had lived for many years. I had just the strength to say, "Thank you" for this rainbow sign, the promise that God was still with Becky and me.

In the weeks that followed, I was impressed to find that Becky was less afraid of dying than of being haunted by her old, angry self. One day when I met her at Queen's, I was surprised to find Becky in tears. We had planned for her to begin a palliative radiation treatment for a painful tumor that had appeared in one hip, and afterward attend the art class, which sometimes was held in the lobby of the radiology department and sometimes at an outdoor lanai shaded by trees. Becky was looking forward to the class, but said she was depressed because she'd been snapping and yelling at her caregivers. She feared that "the old Becky" was back.

I told her it was normal to feel anxious about her cancer and that the fact that she was able to name "the old Becky" meant that "the new Becky" was in charge. She perked up a bit and asked if we could stop at the cancer center to see Yoda, the therapy dog. He was available that day, and I said a silent prayer of thanks.

In her book *The Mysterious Lands*, about the deserts of the American Southwest, naturalist Ann Haymond Zwinger relates a fact that runs counter to common wisdom, that in the desert, dryness promotes the formation of flower buds. It's a good metaphor for the spiritual life, but it's also reality, a part of God's creation.

The Bible is full of desert stories, and one theme is that it's in the inhospitable desert environment that our relationship with God has the best chance to develop. The last years of Becky's life are evidence that providing for growth in unpromising circumstances is a technique for survival. And it's not mere survival; after a life of hardship Becky was opening herself to loving others and being loved.

Although Becky didn't discuss God before or after her terminal diagnosis, she did talk about family. She revisited happy childhood memories and spoke about how much she missed our mom and dad and grandparents.

This made sense to me. As hospice chaplain Kerry Egan writes in her book *On Living*, "People in hospice talk to the chaplain about their families because that is how we talk about God. . . . We don't live our lives in our heads, in theology and theories. We live our lives in our families . . . [and] family is where we first experience love and where we first give it. . . . This crucible of love is where we start to ask big spiritual questions, and ultimately it's where they end."

Our family was a place where Becky knew she belonged. And I'm proud of a niece for so deeply understanding Becky's needs. When she learned she was pregnant, the first person she told, after her husband, was Becky, who immediately phoned me to gloat, saying, "I have a secret to tell. You won't believe it!" Growing up in that big, three-generation household, my niece hadn't forgotten how much any gesture of inclusion meant to Becky.

"I HAVE THE CUTEST DOCTOR, AND HE *SURFS!*"

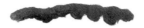

I WAS STILL CONTENDING with anger over Becky's terminal diagnosis, but her good spirits lifted me out of my funk. At one art class after Becky had learned that her cancer was terminal, she described her oncologist by saying, "I have the cutest doctor," adding, "and he *surfs!*" I was delighted to discover that a vestige of the boy-obsessed girl was still in her. As I continued to accompany her to radiation treatments, to movies, to Sunday services at my church, and the art class, Becky acted with courage. Instead of retreating into herself, she reached out to anyone who crossed her path. In the journals I found after her death, Becky was asking questions like, "Why did it have to be me?" But when I was with her not once did she demonstrate any self-pity.

I thought of this during a conversation with one of Becky's cancer center nurses. "It was always a pleasure to see her," she said, adding that they work with many patients whose fears and anxieties make them treat the nursing staff with anger and resentment. "But Becky," she said, "once she became acquainted with us and realized that this was a safe place for her, was so happy and gregarious that she became a people magnet." She added, "There was no pretense with her, no hidden agenda. She was selfless."

The word *selfless* stopped me cold, as Becky had been neurotically selfish and self-absorbed for much of her life. It was a defense that had served her well, but it made the transformation she had undergone in her later years feel miraculous. As she aged, Becky became more genuinely interested in other people. Her personality became more like that of our father, who regarded any stranger as a potential friend.

For both Dad and Becky, the more dire their circumstances, the more they were determined to establish good connections with other people. When he was being treated for aplastic anemia, Dad gave the nurses movie passes at Christmas. And Becky insisted on converting routine medical treatments into meaningful encounters. Oncology nurses doing a blood draw are not used to being asked, "What drew you into this job?" "How long have you been a nurse; have you always worked with cancer patients?" But Becky was relentless, determined to create a friend, a person she could hug when they met again.

COMMUNION

BECKY WAS USING A WHEELCHAIR when she attended church with me at St. Clement's. Where I placed her depended on her mobility; if she could transfer from the chair to a pew, I helped her take a seat, folded the wheelchair, and stored it on a nearby lanai. If she had to stay in the chair, I placed her in a side aisle.

One Sunday my sister was weaker than usual but in a good mood. She had just begun to experience a loss of appetite and difficulty breathing, but happily posed for photos before church with her friend Father Michael. She was not strong enough to stand, so she sat in her wheelchair on an aisle.

After the service Becky was in tears. She told me a woman who was leading her children forward to receive Communion had complained that her wheelchair was taking up too much room in the aisle. And the ushers were too distracted to remind the priest to bring us the Eucharist.

Nothing was going right that morning. After the service I wheeled Becky down the ramp and instead of heading to the parish hall for the regular after-church gathering, I steered her onto the preschool playground where a fair was taking place with live music, games for children, and a potluck lunch. I thought Becky would enjoy this, but she complained that the music was too loud. I moved her farther away from the band and got her a plate of food.

As we were eating, a woman, a retired teacher, stopped to say hello. She is one of our lay eucharistic ministers, commissioned to take Communion to shut-ins. When I told her we hadn't been offered the

Eucharist in church, she asked if we'd like to receive it. We said yes, and she went to the sacristy for the necessary items. Becky set her lunch aside, and I held a Book of Common Prayer so we could read our part of the service together. In the midst of the merriment around us, the laughter of children, the conversation of people visiting over food, we received Communion.

Afterward Becky thanked the woman but said that the noise of the crowd was bothering her. She asked me to take her to the parish house to wait with her for the Handi-Van. By the next Sunday she was dead.

"I HATE MY SYMPTOMS"

ON MONDAY WHEN I MET Becky's Handi-Van at Queen's, I told her I thought that she could no longer handle radiation treatment and going to a movie on the same day. But I'd be happy to take her to movies when she had nothing else planned. Becky grumbled but was realistic about these new limitations. She said to a nurse, "I hate my symptoms." The nurse replied, "I hate your symptoms too."

A few days later Becky said she was tired after her treatment, but she still wanted to attend the art class. A radiation technician had come to the waiting room that morning to tell me that the exertion of transferring her from her wheelchair to the treatment table had given Becky a coughing fit that was the worst they had seen. I thanked him and told him Becky had been complaining that it was harder for her to catch her breath, and while that frightened us she'd always been able to recover.

After the class, Becky was feeling good enough to eat most of a container of yogurt from the hospital cafeteria and give me a list of new films she'd seen advertised and wanted to see. The treatments were due to end soon, and I promised to take her to a movie on the day after they were finished. As she was being wheeled into the Handi-Van, I said, "Love you; see you tomorrow," and she replied, "Love you too." That was our last exchange.

TO GOD'S KINGDOM

My phone rang close to midnight. It was Becky's caregiver, who said that as she was getting my sister ready for bed, she'd had a coughing fit and stopped breathing. Becky was now in an ambulance on her way to an emergency room. When I arrived, a young doctor told me my sister was near death, and I told him that dying now was the best thing that could have happened to her. Becky was barely able to squeeze my hand when I took her hands in mine. But I believe she heard me when I told her that I loved her and was proud of her.

I phoned Father Michael, and after he arrived, the staff asked for a moment to prepare Becky's body, removing the breathing tube they'd inserted in trying to save her life. I had provided Becky's caregivers with an advance directive form that included a do-not-resuscitate order that should have gone with Becky in the ambulance. But they had neglected to give it to the EMTs, which meant that they had attempted to revive her. I was sad Becky had to endure that, but also grateful that the crew's efforts had not succeeded. If they had been able to bring Becky back, she might have suffered more brain damage from a lack of oxygen, erasing her forceful, sassy personality.

Father Michael and I were given a room where we could be alone with Becky. I held her hand, and not knowing if she could hear us, we recited the Twenty-Third Psalm and said the Lord's Prayer. The staff had neglected to remove the stickers that a technician had put on her body as markers before her first radiation treatment. As I peeled them off, I told Becky I remembered that the man had asked her to choose the color of the stickers, and I wasn't surprised that the ones she selected were bright purple.

We stayed with Becky awhile, and after her body was taken to the hospital morgue, I suggested going to a twenty-four-hour bakery and diner a block away. This place, a beloved Honolulu institution, is far off the tourist track, and when two people arrive at three in the morning and one of them is in a clerical collar, the busy waiters know it's serious. They didn't rush us.

We sat at the counter, ordered coffee, and watched in stunned silence as plates laden with huge helpings of food came out of the kitchen. A parade of *loco moco*s: two scoops of white rice, two hamburger patties topped by a fried egg and beef gravy, accompanied by macaroni salad. I couldn't help thinking it was good to have a hospital nearby.

Michael ordered a short stack of pancakes. I wasn't sure I could eat but ordered a piece of cornbread. As I was putting butter on it, I became aware of the boisterous conversations around us. Irritated, I wondered, *Why are these people being so loud?* And then, in my stupor, I realized these folks had been partying and were trying to sober up. I suddenly felt blessed by these amiable strangers, grateful to them for reminding me of the way life goes on, a block from a hospital where people are born and where people die. It wasn't about me or my sister but the present moment, sitting vigil at the Liliha Bakery with a ragtag bunch of human beings, all of us mortal, all of us headed to God's kingdom.

"SHE WAS STILL ABLE TO BE HERSELF"

A DIAGNOSIS OF TERMINAL CANCER sends people into a desert. But one message of the desert stories in the Bible is that God will do the impossible in order to provide for his people. And we are called to recognize the gift that is set before us. We are called—and often challenged—to be grateful.

I had doubted in God's providence, but there it was, like manna. And it was enough. Becky had been granted a quick death; her symptoms hadn't troubled her for long. She had been happy up to the end, complaining just a few hours before her death that I hadn't taken her to a movie in over a week. At Becky's funeral, when I told this to a cancer center nurse, she said, "Oh, that's good—she was still able to be herself."

Cynics and skeptics might protest that this is just one dramatic example and proof of nothing: What if Becky had entered hospice and endured more dreaded decline? I have just enough faith to answer that if God's providence hadn't come in the form it did, it would have come in another.

A recurring phrase in the Psalms speaks of offering "a sacrifice of praise." That use of the word "sacrifice" seemed odd to me when I first heard it. How is praise a sacrifice? But now I believe that there are many circumstances in which praising and giving thanks means that we're not clinging to what we wanted but accepting what life has handed us. It's not positive thinking, or looking "on the bright side." It's a realism than can endure deep darkness and detect the grace that exists even in distressing circumstances. It's up to us to recognize such grace and open our hearts to receive it. Our great consolation is knowing that God is present wherever we are, even when we're walking in a desert, in the shadow of death. Becky believed this to her dying day.

TULIPS

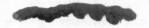

THE DAY AFTER BECKY DIED, Father Michael and I picked up her possessions at her care home. They fit into three cardboard boxes and two shopping bags. We went to the church, where I could sort through the items at a large table in the parish hall. I had to work fast, as a group would need the table within the hour. I was grateful for the time constraint, as it forced me to concentrate on the task at hand.

A rush of memories came as I sorted through Becky's things. In her last years she'd lived in one small room but had found space for one of our family Christmas photographs that someone, probably our dad, had put in a box-like frame for her so it could stand on her dresser. It was taken when Becky still lived with the family; our oldest nieces were teenagers and our younger niece and nephew were in elementary school. Becky stands next to me in the center of the photo wearing a blue muumuu and a big smile.

I found a stack of Becky's journals, which I'd not seen before, and also the many Nancy Drew mysteries I had bought her. There was also the first Harry Potter book, which she never finished, telling me it was too difficult. There was a copy of *The Great Gatsby*, the last book I'd given her. She'd asked for it after seeing the previews for the Leonardo DiCaprio film. When I asked her how she liked the book, she said that her favorite scene was the party, and beamed with pride when I told her that it was one of the most famous party scenes in literature.

There was a great pile of fashion magazines. Becky was ungainly, but she enjoyed reading magazines like *Elle* and *Glamour*. *Marie Claire* was a favorite, and I'd gotten her a subscription. Her clothing was mostly items the family had provided on Becky's birthdays and at Christmas. One niece remembers that she enjoyed watching Becky open her gifts, as she "seemed so excited to receive the simplest thing. She liked pretty things. Pretty shirts. Pretty makeup. Pretty socks. There was always so much color to her."

Becky was hard on her clothing and tended to keep wearing items she liked until they fell apart. That's one thing we had in common; when I was a teenager my mother often complained about me wearing the same dress over and over. As she did the family laundry, I've long suspected that Mom gave clothes she was tired of seeing a little rip that would grow as the washing machine spun them around.

Years of having her clothes washed in group home machines had left many of Becky's items too ratty to be donated. Still, Becky's personality shone through. Some dresses were ridiculously loud: a turquoise-and-purple leopard print threaded with gold for good measure; a gauze dress that constituted an orange, green, yellow, and red extravaganza. Becky craved bling, so there were caps and jackets decorated with studs and fake jewels. The newest item was a flannel robe I had bought for her. Her last care home had been in upper Kalihi Valley, where the trade winds coming over the Koolau mountains can be chilly, and during her cancer treatments she had complained about being cold.

There was the quilt our mother had received on retiring from teaching in 1987, each individual square of the patchwork made by a fellow teacher or grateful parent. I had found it in the closet of my mother's apartment a few weeks after she moved into the nursing home wing of her senior living facility. It had been on her bed when she died, and afterward I gave it to Becky.

At the bottom of the last box, under the quilt, were items I'd never seen but evidently mattered to Becky, as she had managed to hold on to them during many moves over the years. A diploma from San Marcos High School in Santa Barbara, dated January 1972, when Becky would have been seventeen, and small certificates from the Devereux School that my father had put into cheap frames for her. The plastic covers were now cracked and cloudy, but words on the yellowed paper attested to Becky's accomplishments, "Devereux Awards" for citizenship, for modern dance, for improvement in personal hygiene, for serving on the student council, printed in Gothic lettering and duly signed by school officials. One read simply, "Tulips."

"I AM THE BUTTERFLY, SPREAD THE WINGS"

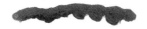

IN READING BECKY'S JOURNALS, I was reminded again of how skilled she was at expressing herself in a terse, dry style that provided an amusing and accurate picture of herself and others. One day, on a page titled "Keeping track of my moods," she wrote: "Kathy comes and we both hyper. Mom deal with it. We go to a movie."

In just a few words she conveys a lifetime of anguish: "Think about how I was born and became special. Feel a little better after talk to mom, the ugly duck in our family. I got wet as a duck today walking home from the bus stop in the rain."

In notes she was preparing for a social worker, she wrote: "Kathy and I too similar in mental health, alike like twins. But I am the butterfly, spread the wings. I am more sociable than the bookworm."

Butterfly to bookworm: what a writer she was. What a writer she might have been.

"TABITHA, GET UP"

MY SISTER DIED EARLY on a Thursday morning; the next Sunday I was scheduled to be a lector at church. As we were in the Easter season, the first reading was from the book of Acts, the story of a woman named Tabitha, renowned for skill as a weaver and also for her many acts of charity. She has died, and her friends have prepared her body for burial. They send for the apostle Paul and ask that he pray over her and say a blessing. When he arrives, these friends do what we do when we mourn our dead: they talk about her, they show him the beautiful cloth she had woven. Alone with the body, Paul says, "Tabitha, get up." The woman opens her eyes and sits up. Taking her by the hand, he shows her friends that she is still alive.

I told Father Michael I wasn't sure that I could read that story on Sunday. The reading had made me wonder why I didn't try that in the emergency room and say, "Becky, get up!" Michael said I didn't have to decide right away; I could think about it, and even at the last minute, on Sunday morning, if I felt I couldn't do it, he'd find someone else.

I practiced the reading at home, stumbling through my first attempts, unable to finish. The more I practiced, the easier it became to read without weeping. By Sunday I had come to feel that it was important for me to read that passage because it was about a resurrection, and in telling it I could honor Becky's resurrection story. The Bible is like that, a friend who speaks hard truths, challenging us but offering consolation when we need it most. It has the power to remove even the heavy stone from a grieving heart.

As my sister approached the age of sixty, she had finally figured out that for people to like her, all she had to do was be herself. She had changed so much that I doubt people who knew her as a conniving, angry, and belligerent young woman would have recognized her. She'd gone from harboring a load of rage to someone whose primary virtue was gratitude. That feels like resurrection to me.

THE PERFECT THING TO SAY

MY SISTER CHARLOTTE AND I were at the funeral home giving a staff member information about Becky. We'd provided the basics, her dates of birth and death, the names of next of kin. When the woman asked, "What did she do?" I was at a loss but my sister spoke up: "Put down artist," which was the perfect thing to say.

It was also a blessing, because from the time she was a child, Charlotte had an exceptionally contentious relationship with Becky. When Charlotte spoke those three words, I felt the presence of the Holy Spirit in all its power as Advocate, Counselor, Consoler, Helper, and Intercessor. As it breathed new life into that dreary, death-haunted room, I was reassured to learn that after all the turmoil and anguish Becky's behavior had caused my sister, what remained was love.

LIKE A CHILD AT HOME

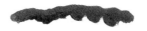

FOR BECKY'S FUNERAL I selected Scripture readings around the themes of reassurance and home. One psalm, 84, speaks of coming to God's dwelling place and finding that "the sparrow herself finds a home, and the swallow a nest" (v. 4 Grail). Our reading from the eighth chapter of Paul's letter to the Romans reminded us that nothing can separate us from the love of God. I chose a hymn, a magnificent rendering of Psalm 23 by Isaac Watts, "My Shepherd Will Supply My Need," because it ends promising that God will one day welcome us "like a child at home." Because of Becky's love for angels, I chose the version of an ancient Gregorian chant, the "In paradisum" that's in the Episcopal hymnal. It begins, "May choirs of angels lead you to paradise."

I was struck by the variety of people who attended Becky's funeral: Mrs. R., who no one in the family had seen for many years; a retired judge who had been a classmate of my brother from his undergraduate years at the University of Hawaii; several of Becky's oncology nurses. One, Yoda's handler, said she'd almost brought the dog as well but wasn't certain if he'd be allowed in the church. I told her he would have been welcome, and it would have pleased Becky to know that she had thought about bringing him.

Becky's counselor and internist from Kōkua Kalihi Valley both came, and the family Becky had lived with for the past four years, after she entered adult foster care, also came. Their adult children and young grandchildren came as well, kids who affectionately called Becky "Auntie B." St. Clement's was full not only of parish members but also with people from her art class and many of the people Becky had befriended at the senior living facility where our parents had spent their last years.

At the reception after Becky's funeral, we used the parish hall again to display her paintings. John, in his eulogy, said of Becky's art that it was her last gift to us.

With the memorial money we received in honor of Becky, the family made donations to the Queen's Cancer Center art class and Kōkua Kalihi Valley. The clinic used the money to buy a beautiful wooden table, chairs, shelving, and lamps for an unused room in their basement. They now have meetings there, and staff members go there when they need some quiet time to themselves. One of Becky's paintings hangs on the wall.

"IT WAS LIKE SHE TOOK ALL THE LIGHT WITH HER"

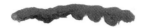

I RETURNED TO THE CANCER CENTER art class a week after Becky died, to finish her last project, making luggage tags for family members. I made one for myself as well, and flight attendants and other passengers often ask me if the photograph on the tag is of myself as a child. It's a classic black-and-white school photograph from the early 1960s of a little girl with a lopsided but endearing smile. She's wearing a blouse with a Peter Pan collar. Her hair is shiny, having been washed for the occasion. She seems slightly amused by the proceedings, expectant and happy.

I tell people that the photo is of my sister who died, and now she travels with me. It's of Becky at the age of six, before all the problems, before all the medications, before anger began to harden that sweet face.

I didn't expect to return to the art class again, but several years after Becky's death, I received a call from the teacher. She had found some Christmas cards Becky had made and asked if I might like to have them. So I went to the class, and as I approached the group—they were meeting that day on familiar ground, the radiation department—a man stood to greet me. I'll call him Sam.

He'd been in the class with Becky but had missed a number of sessions at the time of Becky's last illness in the spring of 2013. When he returned and Becky was absent, he'd been stunned to learn that she had died. He told me her death had hit him hard, and he hadn't been able to make any art since. He said, "It was like she took all the light with her."

Sam and Becky had made an odd couple. Becky was outgoing and effusive; Sam dignified and reserved. Becky quickly plunged into assignments, but Sam strategized for so long that you wondered if he'd be able to complete his work during class. Becky employed splashes of color; Sam used line and geometric design. Both ended up making beautiful paintings, and he and Becky would sit together and quietly converse.

In trying to articulate what Becky had meant to him, he said, "I saw her. I understood who she was, and I got the feeling that she recognized that." I told him I sensed that Becky had "seen" him as well. I suspected that this was as rare an experience for him as it was for her. But when he called Becky "a woman without guile," I laughed and said that while I knew what he meant, growing up with Becky I'd seen plenty of guile in action. I added that in her later years, after she'd contended with two bouts of cancer, much of that had vanished.

Sam told me that it had been at least a year since he'd attended the class and marveled that I happened to be there on the day he had decided to return. Having no idea about Sam's religious beliefs, I ventured to say that I felt this was the Holy Spirit in action. He nodded and said, "I won't argue with that."

BECKY'S BIRDS

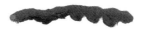

DURING THE LAST YEARS of my sister's life, when she had few joys to sustain her, she took great pleasure in observing the small white birds flitting about the trees at Queen's Hospital. Whether she was watching them through a window of a hospital room or waiting for the Handi-Van, it was a good day for us if those birds came into view.

I discovered that they are white terns, or "fairy" terns, the term my sister preferred. I told Becky that the name had likely been bestowed on them because of their delicate features and the way they dart, swoop, and play in the air. But to her these were magical birds from a magical place. The Hawaiian name for white fairy terns is *manu-o-Kū*, and legend describes them as the birds that guided the Polynesians north in their discovery of the Hawaiian Islands. They are one of the few native birds that have adapted well to the urban environment of Honolulu. I would tell Becky when I saw them elsewhere in town; I once had spotted six of them flying around the family's former home in Mānoa Valley.

These birds do seem magical, flying closely together as if in a synchronized dance. I see the birds nearly every day, and still think of them as Becky's birds.

THE GOSPEL ACCORDING TO REBECCA

AFTER BECKY DIED, I looked up the word *gospel* in the *Oxford English Dictionary*. I knew that it translates as "good news," but I learned that in its long history it has also meant that which is true, an account of the events of Jesus' life, and something that can act as a guide. That "good" part still nagged at me, and I wondered if there were a way to convey that "good" doesn't come neatly packaged as something pleasant. It can mean enduring hard times with only a shred of hope to lead you, a hint of light in one's bleakest moments. I began to wonder what sort of gospel my sister would have written at the end of her life:

> It's a tough gospel, not an easy one. The good is there, but hiding. The devil has some of the best lines, like at the beginning of Genesis, and I've strayed far from the garden, walking through a desert bearing ugly names: perinatal hypoxia, bipolar syndrome, post-traumatic stress disorder. Tempted by rage, I allowed it to define me. Flashbacks and nightmares often woke me; I rose angry every morning. It hurt to know that the agony I suffered all my life was preventable. Careless people had cursed me with their mistakes.
>
> Hope is scant; I've been walking this brutal wasteland for nearly sixty years. But people have also been a blessing. Throughout my journey, when so many mocked and spurned me, there were always those who cared, who helped me find freedom from torment. Not many, but a few: teachers, friends, coworkers. Doctors who saved my life on

more than one occasion. Counselors and social workers who made me feel safe but also challenged me to improve my behavior. People in church who didn't complain if I sang too loudly or out of tune. So many who offered hugs, and many who gladly received them. Above all there was family—my parents, my brother and Marilyn, sisters, nieces and a nephew—offering love that was steadfast and sure.

I received much good guidance from Joyce, and the drugs that helped me cope with my bipolar disorder. I needed all of that, but I also needed transformation, something that therapy and medication can point to, but only Christ can provide.

I believe that God's great warrior, the Archangel Michael, whose image I carried for years, fought alongside me as I fought through life. For many years I did battle every day. But there came a time when I didn't have to fight anymore; I was thankful just to be alive.

I think of the angels in their terrifying aspect, who no longer frighten me, the angels sent into wheat fields at harvest to burn away the weeds and gather the grain. I do feel gathered, as if much of what was bad in me has been destroyed in a purifying fire. The old Becky, who wasted so much time harboring jealousy, resentment, and rage, is gone. What remains is gratitude. It overwhelms me, and I'm constantly thanking people for any little thing they do for me. I used to do this so people would like me and give me what I wanted, but now I'm thankful in a different way. Gratitude lights my path, which has become less stony and rough. There are fewer bushes whose thorns hamper my passage, and I walk freely. One day a woman at church said to me, "Becky, you live thanksgiving." I can't explain it.

They read from John's Gospel at my funeral, and Jesus said, "I will not leave you orphaned." I have come to believe that his words are true. It's a new feeling, to not worry anymore about being cast out and forgotten. Instead there is the great promise of the new heavens *and the new earth in the Revelation. One day I will be a bride adorned for her bridegroom. A secret husband no more, he will be with me for all the world to see. I believe in the good news, words I first heard as a child but only now have come to recognize as the truth that has set me free: "God himself will be with them . . . ; he will wipe every tear from their eyes."*

"AND I WILL RAISE THEM UP"

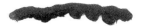

A FEW MONTHS AFTER my sister's death I was asked to preach at an Episcopal church in New England. The lectionary provided two classic resurrection stories: Elijah asking God to restore an impoverished widow's son to life, and Jesus, on encountering another widow whose only son has died, having compassion on her and saying, "Young man, I say to you, arise." And he does.

As I was preaching during the Easter season, it was difficult not to reflect that while the stone from Jesus' tomb had been removed, one remained firmly lodged in my grieving heart. In my sermon I talked about my sister Rebecca and how much I missed her, telling the congregation about her life and how glad I was that she had died a blessed person; despite her cancer she was happier than she'd been in years.

This church has an unusual architecture; the sanctuary is nearly round, with the pulpit and altar in the middle of the wooden pews. This gives congregational singing an added resonance, and as we sang one hymn, "I Am the Bread of Life," its words affected me deeply. The refrain is from the Gospel of John: "And I will raise them up, and I will raise them up, and I will raise them up on the last day." As we sang these phrases repeatedly, the organ louder with each verse, I began to feel that something had changed. Within me, within this small congregation, and within the world, belief in the impossible was suddenly possible. Through the voices of everyone singing, the words had come to life and Becky was with us, blessing us all.

IRON MAN 3

AFTER BECKY'S FUNERAL my brother suggested that we take her ashes to *Iron Man 3*. I had seen the first two Iron Man movies with her, and she enjoyed them immensely, happily declaring them to be "action packed." That was Becky's catch phrase for any movie containing a surfeit of fights, gunfire, car chases, and explosions. She had probably heard "action packed" once in a movie trailer, and it stuck.

This was typical of Becky; once she found a word that suited her, she used it for years. "Special" was another one. She had been labeled "stupid," "slow," "retarded," "developmentally disabled," and when the phrase "special education" came into use, she seized on it. "Special" was a word she was glad to claim. She used it with people she was meeting for the first time, if she thought they might expect too much from her, as they often did.

I remember very little of that third Iron Man film, except for the satisfaction of holding the box of Becky's ashes close to my heart and thinking how much she would have loved the movie. She would have been glad to see one of her nieces sitting next to me, pregnant with her second child. And if I could tell Becky that we had taken her ashes straight from her funeral to the theater, I'm sure she would say, "Of course you did. I'm special."

ACKNOWLEDGMENTS

I'M GRATEFUL TO MY FAMILY for their support, and especially my parents who kept the many letters Becky wrote to them over the years. I want to thank the staff of the Queens Hospital Cancer Center and am grateful to everyone at Kōkua Kalihi Valley, especially Flo Baldonado and Laura C. DeVilbiss; the care they offered my sister was a lifesaver. I deeply appreciate their granting me access to Becky's complete medical files after her death. I had many of Becky's words from her letters. But reading what she said to her counselor and physician at the clinic, and what emergency room physicians said about her condition on the many occasions when she went to them for help, were invaluable in the writing of this book.

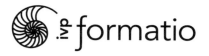

BECOMING OUR TRUE SELVES

The nautilus is one of the sea's oldest creatures. Beginning with a tight center, its remarkable growth pattern can be seen in the ever-enlarging chambers that spiral outward. The nautilus in the IVP Formatio logo symbolizes deep inward work of spiritual formation that begins rooted in our souls and then opens to the world as we experience spiritual transformation. The shell takes on a stunning pearlized appearance as it ages and forms in much the same way as the souls of those who devote themselves to spiritual practice. Formatio books draw on the ancient wisdom of the saints and the early church as well as the rich resources of Scripture, applying tradition to the needs of contemporary life and practice.

Within each of us is a longing to be in God's presence. Formatio books call us into our deepest desires and help us to become our true selves in the light of God's grace.

LIKE THIS BOOK?

Scan the code to discover more content like this!

Get on IVP's email list to receive special offers, exclusive book news, and thoughtful content from your favorite authors on topics you care about.

IVPRESS.COM/BOOK-QR